fighting
the
freshman
fifteen

fighting
the
freshman
fifteen

A COLLEGE WOMAN'S GUIDE TO
GETTING REAL ABOUT FOOD AND
KEEPING THE POUNDS OFF

ROBYN FLIPSE, M.S., R.D.
with Marisa and Marchelle Bradanini

 THREE RIVERS PRESS · NEW YORK

To my parents, Peter and Joan Flipse,
who saw five daughters through
college in good spirits and great shape.
—Robyn Flipse

Marchelle and Marisa would like to dedicate
this book to their parents, Michael and Sherry Bradanini.

Published by Three Rivers Press, New York, New York.
Member of the Crown Publishing Group, a division of Random House, Inc.

www.randomhouse.com

THREE RIVERS PRESS and the Tugboat design are registered trademarks of Random House, Inc.

Printed in the United States of America

Design by Rhea Braunstein

Library of Congress Cataloging-in-Publication Data
Flipse, Robyn.
    Fighting the freshman fifteen: a college woman's guide to getting real about food and keeping the pounds off / by Robyn Flipse, with Marisa and Marchelle Bradanini.
    1. Weight loss. 2. College freshmen—Health and hygiene. 3. Women college students—Health and hygiene. 4. Nutrition. I. Bradanini, Marisa. II. Bradanini, Marchelle. III. Title.
RM222.2.F538 2002
613.2—dc21   2002022929

ISBN 0-609-80960-1

10 9 8 7 6 5 4 3 2 1
First Edition

acknowledgments

I owe thanks to all of the young women who have sought my help after encountering the freshman fifteen while away at college for the first time. They taught me some lessons that weren't covered in my nutrition education. The challenges they faced and conquered provided the wisdom I needed to write this book.

—*Robyn Flipse*

We thank our parents, Michael and Sherry Bradanini, for their continual support and for teaching us to strive for our passions in life.

—*Marisa and Marchelle Bradanini*

contents

introduction

G ET out your highlighting markers, a notepad, and a pen and turn down the music, girls, because you've got some serious studying to do here. If you're the least bit concerned about gaining the freshman fifteen, then this book is required reading for you.

Your course instructors are not the usual stodgy professors who haven't left their cluttered offices in decades. We are a practicing registered dietitian with twenty-five-plus years of experience counseling young women just like you and two college girls who are sisters. One went through the horror of gaining the freshman fifteen, then figured out a way to repair her pudgy body by preparing her own food in the confines of her dorm room and making smarter choices when she ventured out. The other, her kid sister, followed the meal plans and made the recipes her big sister created when she eventually arrived on campus so that she wouldn't have to endure even one pound of the fated fifteen. Together they have amassed all the "before and after" lessons you need to learn so that you don't repeat them in your first year, too.

It is important to note that the freshman fifteen was not a chapter in any nutrition text I ever studied as an aspiring nutritionist or any lecture I ever attended in my continuing education. But once I was comfortably settled into my practice for about ten years, I started getting frantic calls from the mothers of college girls. It was usually around Thanksgiving time, when the daughters had made their first visit home after eight weeks in college. The moms were concerned about the five to ten pounds their daughters had already gained.

The first appointment would be made for the week the daughter was due home for her semester break in December. Then, when she arrived, she was often five pounds heavier than the weight reported during the Thanksgiving call. It was an astounding weight gain, one that had the girl, her mother, and me equally baffled.

The diet histories I have completed for every girl I have counseled during the last fifteen years since encountering those first initiates to the freshman fifteen reveal a common thread. College life is uncharted terrain for each arriving freshman, but no matter which path a girl takes, there will be plenty to eat and drink along the way.

The single biggest change I can identify since my own first year at college twelve hundred miles away from home some thirty years ago is the constant availability of food on campus. The cafeterias are opened continuously now, not just during the rigidly enforced breakfast-lunch-supper hours when I attended. But even if the cafeteria does close at 2:00 P.M. each afternoon or by 8:00 P.M. each night, there are infinite other places to buy food. College campuses are indeed a microcosm of America, with their fast-food outlets, snack bars, coffee shops, and quickie marts all operating twenty-four hours a day.

Dormitory life has changed dramatically as well. Up to the 1960s dorms had very strict curfews, which greatly limited the chances of students slipping out for pizza at midnight. They also ruled out the hope of having a pizza delivered, since only the resident adviser could open the door after curfew.

There were many other "house rules" that served to curb our appetites, too. Hot plates and toaster ovens were prohibited due to the fire and safety hazards they posed; minirefrigerators were disallowed due to the electrical expense incurred to run them. Certainly no one had a microwave oven in her room because they were still quite huge and very expensive to buy at that time.

A row of vending machines in the dorm basement was the closest thing we had to twenty-four-hour food service, but then we rarely had the exact change needed to make a purchase. If we did, all that was often left in the machines were Life Savers and chewing gum.

Gradual policy changes in the late '60s and early '70s set the stage for the earliest appearance of the freshman fifteen. It was during these years that cafeteria hours were extended, outside food services opened concessions on campus, and curfews ended. So freshman girls had ample opportunities to eat!

One more thing occurred that increased the appetites of college girls. Around the mid-1970s, many college dormitories became coed—by hall or by floor. Eating and drinking with the guys opened up a whole new world of calories for the girls. And without a compass to help navigate this very strange and new territory, the path was paved with unwanted pounds.

But now, finally, you have a scout who can mark a new trail for you. There is no need to walk into the wilderness alone and arrive on the other side of the woods heavy and depressed. All you have to do to begin your journey is turn the page.

1

welcome to campus!

J OIN us for an orientation around campus that promises to answer the one question every freshman girl has: "How can I avoid gaining weight during my first year away at college?" We know you have anticipated your first semester with a mixture of joy and fear, and we are prepared to put that fear to rest. Understanding how and why the freshman fifteen happens is half the battle in keeping it from squeezing into your jeans with you by Christmas break.

First, it is essential to recognize that there are really only *three* things that can make you gain weight this semester:

1. Overeating
2. Overdrinking
3. Underdoing

Conquer these, and you'll be forever svelte. But nothing is ever that simple and so we must look even closer at what it is that can lead to the excessive eating, drinking, and insufficient activity that define college life for most freshman girls. Pay very close attention to the following lessons, because they may be the most valuable ones you'll learn this term.

Too Much Freedom

For most of you, this is the first time in your life that you can literally come and go as you please. You no longer have to answer to a parent, teacher, or any other adult about what you're doing, who you're doing it with, or if you're dressed appropriately. No one cares whether you've made your bed, finished your classwork, or eaten some breakfast. You are on your own.

Gaining all of this freedom so suddenly takes some time getting used to. Many of you will try to find your way by testing the limits of your liberation. You'll stay out very late at night, sleep very late into the morning, and eat at odd hours just to see if anyone notices. And what you'll quickly realize is, no one does.

Once you are really convinced there are no rules to govern your personal conduct and no enforcers even if there were, your common sense seems to disappear and hedonism takes over. Do you remember reading *Lord of the Flies* in high school? Everything and anything that was once forbidden or denied can now be indulged. A whole box of Pop-Tarts and a tube of Pillsbury biscuits becomes breakfast. Eating pizza at midnight every night is the norm. Some days nothing but chocolate and coffee are consumed.

You may also recall that in *Lord of the Flies* the ending wasn't pretty. Too much freedom is *not* a good thing. Just like those British schoolboys let loose on a desert island, you, too, must rein in your impulses if you have any hope of remaining civilized. Civilized people do not eat one-pound bags of Doritos all by themselves. They share them with at least eleven other people so that you can each have just one and one-third ounces, or about 200 calories apiece. It's the only fair way to do battle with the freshman fifteen.

Too Much Food

Then there is the little matter of the prepaid dining card. Eating from an all-you-can-eat buffet at every meal is like holding a one-way ticket to the freshman fifteen if you don't retain some self-control. In your college cafeteria you will face endless quantities of bagels, pasta, frozen yogurt, muffins, French fries, and chocolate chip cookies and you may take all you want. Your mother is not going to be at the end of the line to check your tray and make sure you also took a piece of fruit and some protein to balance your meal. How about a carton of milk with that Cap'n Crunch? Truth is, you can eat nothing but carbs morning, noon, and night, but if you do, the freshman fifteen will soon follow.

Your best hope here is to look at your tray after you've been to all of the food stations but before you check out, then ask yourself: "Does this look like a meal my mother would approve of?" If the answer isn't a resounding "Yes," then you must return some of those empty calories and replace them with foods your mom or another significant other would approve of. There's no doubt about it, self-control is much easier to practice when a second pair of eyes are on you.

Too Many Parties

Even if you find the food detestable in the cafeteria and are wasting five hundred dollars a month on a meal plan you never use, there is still the matter of college parties. Any time of day, for any reason at all, people are ready to have a good time on campus. This isn't at all like high school, where you had to wait for the weekend and hope that someone's parents were out of town to find a good party. More beer than you ever imagined is available, literally all the time, somewhere on or around campus.

But, alas, too much of a good thing usually turns bad, and all that drinking will definitely add to your girth if you're not careful. Try to think of each can of beer as two slices of bread—both have about 150 calories. Every six-pack you put away is close to eating a *loaf* of bread! Or imagine each glass of punch or blender drink as a big scoop of premium ice cream worth about 300 calories. After two or three of these drinks, you're into hot-fudge-sundae territory with whipped cream on top. How many of those do you think you can get away with eating in a night? In a week?

When it comes to parties, it may help to imagine that your dad is watching you pump that keg. If that isn't a Kodak moment you'd like to share, find some seltzer to keep the freshman fifteen at bay.

Too Much Strangeness

While college is supposed to be a time of discovery and an immersion into an independent and almost-adult world, all this newness can also feel threatening. It can really hit home when you wake up that first morning in the dorm and realize you are living with strangers. From the moment you received your acceptance letter, the pressure was on: You were going to have to make all new friends because your old high school buddies were not going with you on this adventure.

Even once you're settled into your dorm room, the newness of college life isn't over. You've got to read a map just to find out where to buy stamps, make color copies, get some cough medicine, or buy a birthday card for your little sister.

That's when it may strike you, as it did Dorothy when she landed in Oz, that you're "not in Kansas anymore."

As if all that wasn't frustrating enough, you still have to figure out where all your classes are, or where they've been relocated to, and decide where the best place around town is to buy the new or used books you'll need for each one. You need to track down all the ATMs within a one-mile radius of campus, find a decent place to get your hair cut, and remember to save all your quarters if you have any intention of doing your laundry.

When it all seems just too strange to bear, one of the first things most freshmen turn to for reassurance is comfort food. You know, those familiar tastes and smells that let you believe that all is still safe and secure in your world. Things like macaroni and cheese, mashed potatoes and gravy, pancakes and syrup, and butterscotch pudding with whipped cream on top can really make you feel at home. Unfortunately, if you find

---

☀ MARISA:
When I lived at home, I always took the healthy, home-cooked meals we had for granted. It was a real shock when I got to college and didn't have anyone looking over my shoulder and telling me what to eat or fixing healthy meals for me.

☀ MARCHELLE:
I found that most college students are so happy to move away from home, they wind up eating all of the things their parents told them not to while growing up. When you live together in a dorm, it's very difficult not to just go along with everyone else and order that pepperoni pizza. . . .

yourself seeking solace from these emotionally rewarding foods just a bit too often, they will stay with you in the form of the freshman fifteen long after you've found your way around campus.

Too Many Choices

Another equally powerful force that may push you toward a monotonous lineup of high-caloric foods at each meal is the outrageous selection of unfamiliar foods on sale in the cafeteria. Some days you may feel as if you're attending college in another country, the foods being served look so unusual to you. Things like frittata (Italian omelet), feijoada (Portuguese stew), and fattoush (Arabian mixed salad) are sure to appear. That's when most nimble-minded people go directly for the items they recognize as all-American: cheeseburgers, chicken fingers, and chili dogs. And, of course, a side order of French fries.

You may also seek refuge from foods with strange ingredients by piling your tray with the brand names you've grown to trust in your first eighteen years of eating: Wise, Herr's, Frito-Lay, Nabisco, Sara Lee, and Hershey. Not a good strategy, either.

While there is no need to eat any food you can't relate to until you are good and ready, you may have to take a second look at the cafeteria spread to be sure you don't pass up some of the familiar fare that could help balance out your meals. For example, you'll probably recognize the apples, bananas, and oranges in a big bowl near the cashier's, and the yogurt, chocolate milk, and cheese sticks in the refrigerated case. Did you look closely at the hot-food line for the vegetable soup and the baked potatoes? How about the sliced Swiss cheese and boiled ham at the deli counter? When it comes to fighting the freshman fifteen, being fussy is your prerogative, being stubborn is not.

Too Much Socializing

Sharing food is a uniquely human behavior. It actually separates us from the rest of the animal kingdom, which chooses not to invite other creatures from outside the pack into the den for a bite to eat. But since it is one of *our* favorite ways to socialize, you must be mindful of just how friendly you want to be with every person you meet while at college. Your socializing skills will be enhanced by the fact that the café is always open, care packages from home are viewed as community property, and eating is infinitely more engaging than studying, so there's always someone ready to get acquainted!

This is where getting in touch with some of your suppressed animal instincts will become very useful. Just as animals don't entertain over dinner, they also do not eat more than they need to in order to satisfy their hunger. Even when a wild animal is really hungry and tracks down and slays its favorite beast, it eats only what it needs and leaves the rest for scavengers. It does not eat until it is so stuffed, it wants to vomit. Neither should you.

To keep your "social eating" in check, you will need to cultivate this primitive instinct for hunger control. That means you need to train yourself to always eat when you are hungry and *never* eat when you are not.

Too Few Meals

One of the built-in safeguards against totally irrational eating while you were living at home and going to high school was the unshakable routine. Your alarm rang at the same time every morning to start your day. Then a bell rang at school to tell you when it was time to go to lunch and when it was time to go home. Your parents may have stocked the fridge and cupboards with a lot of healthful, low-fat stuff to snack on, and they may have told you when it was time to come to the table for a dinner of more of the same. As much as you may have hated living under the tyranny of such a schedule, you also couldn't get into too much trouble with innumerable calories, either.

But all that has changed now that you're in college. With any luck, there is some similarity to your Monday-Wednesday-Friday class schedule and the one you follow on Tuesday and Thursday. If not, you probably have no two days that start and end at the same time. Without some kind of structure to your life, meals just seem to fall off the radar screen and an ad-lib feeding plan takes its place. To an experimental lab rat, that means it gets to eat however much it wants, whenever it wants. And although rats are a lower life form and have yet to start socializing with other rats over drinks and hors d'oeuvres, they *can* become fat if given access to too much of the food they like without having to forage for it. And if they get fat on an ad-lib diet, so can you.

Eating regular meals is your only defense against that portion of the freshman fifteen that can be directly attributed to grazing. The calories you don't consume at breakfast, lunch, and supper are more than made up for at all those pitstops you make throughout the day. No matter how wacky your schedule may seem, you have to divide each day into evenly spaced time periods where you plan a time to eat every three to four hours. If you don't, you'd better devise an explanation for your parents as to why you'll need a new wardrobe by second semester!

Too Few Fluids

Remember water? It's that clear, flavorless, calorie-free beverage that comes out of faucets, fountains, and designer bottles. You probably had easy access to all the water you wanted back home when the refrigerator was stocked with it and the school lunchroom had an ample supply for sale. Now it's your job to keep regular rations on hand and make it your beverage of choice at least 8 times a day; otherwise, you're not drinking enough. Sure, you may be taking in plenty of other fluids, but what your body needs to meet its daily requirements is the nonalcoholic, noncaffeinated, unsweetened variety.

This isn't just some dieting tip that has been around so long, everyone has forgotten why 8 glasses a day is recommended. And it isn't simply to fill you up so that you'll eat less food. The reason you need those 64 ounces of water a day is to stay properly hydrated. You'll discover in chapter 10 that your body is made up of 55 to 60 percent water. Every day you lose a big portion of that water through the skin, when you breathe, when you eliminate, and through other metabolic processes. If you don't replace the lost water, none of your bodily systems will function as efficiently as they should. In fact, as little as a 3 percent water loss can lead to dizziness, confusion, and impaired thinking. That certainly won't help your GPA.

But of greater concern to everyone trying to keep the freshman fifteen from catching up with them is the fact that those who do not stay fully hydrated tend to eat more—often because they mistake their sense of thirst for hunger. Don't let those signals get crossed. Just reach for a tall drink of water whenever you feel like eating something and make sure you know where you can fill up again when that glass is empty.

Too Much Access

Fast-food chains, convenience stores, coffee shops, and other cheap eateries of every description are probably within walking distance of the front door of your dorm. In fact, you can't go anywhere without passing by these places. Every undeniable craving and senseless whim you have can be readily satisfied if you have a few dollars in your pocket. What you don't dream up on your own you'll be readily reminded of as you trudge across the commons. You see Chili's familiar neon red pepper in the distance and start salivating for a three-cheese quesadilla. Or you pick up the scent of a fresh batch of Mrs. Fields white chunk macadamia cookies wafting through the union. . . .

It's not easy to pass up all those temptations, but you must try. College towns are not magnets for produce stands and juice bars. And those that are in the vicinity are not using a neon sign to mark their location. They also won't have a concession in every other building on campus. But you need to find out where all of these enterprising natural-food markets are so that you can treat yourself to a juicy, ripe mango when the urge for something sweet hits or indulge in a tangy seaweed salad when your palate needs a surprise.

Just think, you can fight both the fast-food giants and the freshman fifteen with the same effort by spending your money on foods that don't come in Styrofoam containers or are on the same menu 365 days a year. Who knows, if you can get enough of your friends to follow suit, you may see a proliferation of fruit and veggie stands around campus by the time you graduate!

Too Little Activity

Sure, college life is filled with plenty of things to do. There are great independent-film festivals to see and humanitarian causes to join. You can hear a new band playing in some bar every night of the week and rally in front of the administration building for a different cause every day. You can write for the school newspaper, host a jazz program on the college radio station, or run for a seat in student government. Then there are clubs, sororities, and dorm committees with which to fill your free time between classes.

Sadly, none of this counts as exercise and won't take the place of all the physical activity you were getting while in high school. Most likely just walking the halls of your old high school, going up and down the stairs, and taking the mandatory phys ed program helped keep you in shape. If you played on any school or recreational sports teams or went to a gym regularly, you were definitely getting more exercise than you are now. You even got a workout when you participated in pep rallies, car washes, field days, class wars, and other school-spirit events back in high school. But that's all over now, so what are you going to do about it?

Freshman year is as good a time as any to hone your skills in time management. Here is what you have to consider. Your week is made up of 168 hours. You will need about 80 of them for sleeping and 14 for dining and dressing. That leaves 74 hours.

If you're taking 15 credits this semester, you must budget 15 hours a week for lectures and labs. Then most professors will tell you you'll need another 3 hours a week per class to keep up with your course work. That means you'll be spending another 15 hours a week on "homework." If you don't have a job, that leaves 44 hours a week for fun and fitness.

Plan to devote at least 5 hours a week to some form of exercise if you are really serious about avoiding the freshman fifteen. If that doesn't seem possible, you're not managing your time well enough. Stop the excuses and start exercising *now*. Do not stop for the rest of your life.

REMEMBER:

Earning a 4.0 is a great grade point average for any freshman girl to achieve. Putting on a pound a week during your first semester at college is *not*.

2

a 3-credit course in weight control

Course Objective

Upon completion of this course you will be able to make food selections to meet your nutritional, caloric, and social needs while avoiding the famous freshman fifteen.

Prerequisites

If you have already taken a *real* nutrition course or think you know everything there is to know about dieting because you've been on every diet, you are a perfect candidate for this course. You are also eligible to take this class if you haven't a clue about weight control. In fact, knowing a lot of food facts and nutrition science will not keep you from gaining the dreaded freshman fifteen.

Content Objectives

To pass this course, what you *know* is not nearly as important as what you *do*. You actually have to eat differently, or more appropriately, so those fifteen extra pounds don't have a chance of graduating with you. Fortunately, your eating habits are not set in stone. You can change the way you eat with the same ease you change majors. Here's how.

To do what it takes to fight the freshman fifteen, you must remember only two indisputable principles. One, you must control calories. Two, you must control portion sizes. That's it. Just count calories and measure portions and over spring break you'll be able to wear the same bathing suit you wore last summer.

If you're thinking, "I already know the caloric content of all my faves and I know that a serving of frozen yogurt is a half-cup," get over it. As we have already pointed out, it does not matter what you *know* if what you *do* when you pull the lever on the self-serve yogurt machine is take close to 2 cups of the stuff and add an unknown quantity of chocolate sprinkles, then sum it up to be about 100 calories.

In order to do the right things to control the calories and portions that will let you win the fight against the freshman fifteen, you're going to need some new skills. Think of it as being more like learning tennis. You can't just read books about the sport to master it. You've got to get out on the court and swing a racquet to perfect your game.

Requirement I

Follow a daily food plan based on your height and activity level.

Lecture Notes

No matter how complicated the pursuit of a balanced, healthy diet may seem, the toughest math you have to do is just to count, and the most complicated menu planning requires only that you put together three foods at a meal. The rest of the expectations are listed below.

✦ Recognize what types of foods you are eating—or what food groups they belong to. To help with this, you should make it your policy never to eat anything you can't identify or classify.

✦ Choose foods from the different food groups at every meal or snack. Mix them up in any way you want—your stomach does not care how you combine the foods you eat or when.

✦ Do not overconsume foods from any one group or consistently leave out foods from any group. No matter how nutritious a food is, it cannot make you superhealthy if you eat more of it. In fact, if you eat more than you need of anything, it can and will make you fat.

✦ Change your choices from week to week and season to season. There is no reason to believe that the best possible lunch in the world is a turkey sandwich without mayo. It isn't, and it's boring, and it will lead to cravings and bingeing if you don't vary your diet with a ham-and-Swiss or egg salad sandwich once in a while.

✦ Keep track of how many servings you eat each day from the different food groups and how many "extras" you've consumed. (This is where the counting comes in handy.) If you eat more than you should one day, cut back during the next few days to offset the excess. Do not try to starve yourself to set the record straight. It won't work. Starving leads to splurging, which means you'll eat even more than you should have when it's over. If you want to get crazy, exercise for another couple of hours.

✦ Get all the physical activity you've scheduled for yourself, then take advantage of any opportunity to do more.

Remember, no one has ever regretted going back to their high school homecoming game all toned and buffed and looking really hot after being in college for half a semester. Many have missed that event due to the excess baggage they were toting.

✺ *MARCHELLE:*

There is no pill or diet that exists so that you can live off hamburgers and cheesecake. You have to develop your own sense of restraint and discipline!

✺ *MARISA:*

A common lunch for me was a large diet soda, gummy bears, and a bag of chips—no wonder I gained weight! It takes willpower to grab a banana instead of a candy bar.

Assignments

1. Go to the student health center or fitness lab on campus and get a professional measurement of your present height and weight, then record them on the **Baseline Data Chart,** page 17. Do not assume that their scale is inaccurate or the results are wrong because of the clothes you were wearing or the time of day or month you were weighed. Use the numbers you get as your baseline—no substitutions.

2. Use Table 2.1, **Calories per Day for Weight Control,** on page 18 to determine how many calories a day you should consume to maintain your present weight, or to lose weight, with the allotted amount of weekly activity; record that on your baseline data chart.

3. Decide when, where, and how you will get the required physical activity each week based on your class and work schedule, then fill in those blanks on your chart. (More

information on what, how, and how much exercise can be found in chapter 10.)

4. Find the food plan for your caloric allowance outlined in Table 2.2, **Daily Food Plans for Different Calorie Levels,** on page 18 and record the recommended daily servings from each food group on your chart.

5. Combine different foods from Table 2.3, **What's in a Food Group?,** on page 18 and Table 2.4, **Decoding Combination Foods,** on page 19 to get your daily rations.

6. BONUS CREDIT: Use the recipes in chapter 11 for no-brainer foods you can quickly and easily make for yourself. Each recipe includes a breakdown of the food group servings in one portion so that you can't fail.

COMPLETE THIS!

BASELINE DATA CHART

DATE:_____ HEIGHT:_____ WEIGHT:_____ DESIRED WEIGHT:_____

CALORIC ALLOWANCE:

To Maintain Present Weight:_____   To Lose Weight:_____

PLANNED HOURS OF PHYSICAL ACTIVITY PER WEEK:_____

DAY	TIME	PLACE	TYPE OF ACTIVITY
Monday	_____	_____	_____
Tuesday	_____	_____	_____
Wednesday	_____	_____	_____
Thursday	_____	_____	_____
Friday	_____	_____	_____
Saturday	_____	_____	_____
Sunday	_____	_____	_____

DAILY FOOD PLAN:

Grain____ Dairy____ Meat____ Fruit___ Vegetable___ Fat___ Extras___

Table 2.1
CALORIES PER DAY FOR WEIGHT CONTROL*

Height

	<5'2"	5'3"–5'6"	>5'7"
Activity			
2 hours	1200	1400	1600
4 hours	1400	1600	1800
6 hours	1600	1800	2000

* Use these caloric allowances to maintain weight. To lose 1 to 2 pounds per week, use the lowest caloric allowance for your height with the most hours of activity per week.
** Activity = total hours of aerobic and resistance activity per week.

Table 2.2
DAILY FOOD PLANS FOR DIFFERENT CALORIE LEVELS

Calorie Levels

	1200	1400	1600	1800	2000
Food Groups					
Grain	4	4	5	6	6
Dairy	2	2	2	3	3
Meat	2	3	3	3	3
Fruit	2	3	3	3	4
Vegetable	3	3	4	4	5
Fat	2	2	3	3	4
Extras	3	4	4	4	6

Table 2.3
WHAT'S IN A FOOD GROUP?

Grain	Breads, rolls, bagels, cereals, pasta, rice, tortillas, crackers, pretzels, popcorn—all made with minimal fat or sugar
Dairy	Low-fat or fat-free milk, yogurt, and cheese or fortified low-fat soy milk and cheese
Meat	Lean meat, skinless poultry, fish, eggs, soy, nuts, and beans
Fruit	Fresh, frozen, canned, and dried fruit or full-strength juice

Vegetable	Raw or cooked, fresh, frozen, canned, or juiced vegetables
Fats	Spreads, dressings, cooking oils, shortening, fried food
Extras	Sweetened drinks, desserts, candy, greasy snack foods, and alcoholic beverages

---

> ✸ *MARISA:*
>
> *We always had healthy leftovers to snack on at home. But in the dorm it was a different story—I had never been surrounded by so many cakes, cookies, ice cream, chips, and candy before.*
>
> ✸ *MARCHELLE:*
>
> *Having Mom do the grocery shopping and preparing the meals made it easy to be a healthy eater before I went to college. Even if I wanted something crazy, I was limited to what was in the kitchen cabinets—all pretty healthy stuff.*

HIGHLIGHT THIS!

Table 2.4
DECODING COMBINATION FOODS

Combo Food	Amount	Food Groups
Baked ziti	1½ cups	2 Grain, ½ Veg, ½ Dairy
Beef vegetable stew	1 cup	1 Grain, 2 Meat, 1 Veg, 1 Fat
Burrito, beef	1 7" tortilla	1½ Grain, 2 Meat, 2 Fat
bean	1 7" tortilla	3 Grain, 1 Meat, 2 Fat
Caesar salad with croutons	2 cups	2 Veg, ½ Grain, 6 Fat
Cheese pizza	⅛ large pie	2 Grain, 1 Dairy, 1 Fat
Cheese ravioli with tomato sauce	1 cup	1 Grain, 1 Dairy, 1 Veg, 1 Fat

Combo Food	Amount	Food Groups
Chef salad with dressing	1 bowl	3 Veg, 3 Meat, 5 Fat
Chicken noodle soup	1 cup	1 Grain
Chili with meat and beans	1 cup	1 Grain, 2 Meat, 1 Veg, 2 Fat
Chow mein (with meat, no rice)	1 cup	½ Grain, 2 Meat, 1 Veg
Club sandwich	1 sandwich	3 Grain, 4 Meat, 4 Fat
Cream soup	1 cup	1 Grain, 1 Fat
Egg roll	1 4" roll	1 Grain, 1 Meat, 1 Veg, 1 Fat
Eggplant Parmesan	1 cup	1 Grain, 2 Dairy, 1 Veg, 4 Fat
Fish sticks	3 sticks	1 Grain, 1 Meat, 3 Fat
French fries	15 pieces	1 Grain, 1 Fat
French toast	2 slices	2 Grain, 1 Meat, 2 Fat
Fried rice	1 cup	2 Grain, 1 Veg, 2 Fat
Gefilte fish	1 piece, egg size	1 Meat
Hoagie sandwich	1 6" sandwich	4 Grain, 3 Meat, 1 Dairy, 4 Fat
Hummus	¼ cup	½ Grain, 1 Meat, 1 Fat
Kugel, potato or noodle	1 cup	2 Grain, 2 Fat
Macaroni and cheese	1 cup	1½ Grain, 1 Dairy, 2 Fat
Muffin, corn, bran, or blueberry	3" high, 3" wide	2 Grain, 1 Fat
Pea, lentil, or bean soup	1 cup	1½ Grain, 1 Meat, 1 Fat
Pot pies	1 4" diameter	3 Grain, 1 Meat, 5 Fat
Quesadilla, cheese	1 6" tortilla	1 Grain, 1 Dairy, 2 Fat
Refried beans	1 cup	2 Grain, 3 Fat
Sushi (fish on rice)	3 pieces	½ Grain, 2 Meat
Tabbouleh	1 cup	2 Grain, ½ Veg, 1 Fat
Taco with beef, lettuce, tomato, and cheese	1 6" taco shell	1 Grain, 1 Meat, ½ Dairy, 2 Fat

Combo Food	Amount	Food Groups
Vegetable lasagna	3" × 4" piece	1 Grain, ½ Dairy, 1 Veg, 2 Fat
Veggie burger	3" wide, ½" thick	2 Meat, 1 Fat
Wonton soup	2 wontons, 1 cup broth	1 Grain, 1 Fat

Requirement II

Recognize standardized serving sizes for all of the foods and beverages you consume.

Lecture Notes:

✦ Serving sizes used on the nutrition facts panel of a food label are *not* necessarily the same as the recommended food group servings. Use the calories per serving information on the label to adjust the serving size to fit the appropriate group(s).

✦ Restaurant portions *definitely* are not the same as food group servings. Not even close. Your best bet is to split a serving with someone or to always take half back to the dorm for another meal.

✦ The volume of a food when measured in measuring cups does NOT equal its weight in ounces. In other words, a cup of Cheerios weighs only 1 ounce while a cup of cooked oatmeal weighs 9 ounces. Do not try to switch back and forth between volume and weight when determining serving sizes or caloric content. It's one or the other.

✦ When uncertain of the recommended portion size for a food, use a comparable item, like ravioli for pierogi or fried shrimp for shrimp tempura.

✦ Use the recipes in chapter 11 to eliminate the guesswork and have the right stuff in the right amounts every time you eat.

> ✵ *MARCHELLE:*
> *Friends of mine tried to starve themselves as a way to lose weight. I found success in what I call "constant moderation."*
>
> ✵ *MARISA:*
> *One thing I learned in college is that just because a product is low-fat or fat-free doesn't mean that serving size doesn't matter. If you eat an entire 4-ounce bag of fat-free chips, you're still consuming 500 calories. Bottom line: the serving does matter.*

Assignments

1. Determine the capacity and dimensions of all of your eating and drinking utensils and record on the **Eating Utensils Chart,** page 22, to aid in portion control when eating in the dorm.

2. Use the serving-size guidelines in Table 2.5, **Standard Serving Sizes for Food Group Portions,** on page 23 to keep track of the *actual* number of portions you eat from each food group.

3. Estimate the serving size for unfamiliar portions using Table 2.6, **Portion Size Comparisons,** on page 30 to guide you when eating away from the dorm.

FIGURE THIS OUT!

EATING UTENSILS CHART

You can save yourself a lot of time measuring your food if you know what the capacity is of the dishes and glassware you normally use. Fill each of these containers with water (except the flat plates), then measure the volume using a measuring cup. Record on the chart the cups and/or ounces each holds. Then measure the height and width for each using a ruler, including the dishes and plates, and record that on the chart.

	CUPS	OUNCES	DIMENSIONS
Coffee mug			
Tall glass			
Short glass			
Sports/water bottle			
Cereal bowl			
Salad bowl			
Soup bowl			
Dessert dish			
Dinner plate			
Lunch plate			
Bread plate			

COPY AND SHRINK, THEN FOLD AND STORE THIS IN YOUR WALLET FOR EASY REFERENCE.

Table 2.5
STANDARD SERVING SIZES FOR FOOD GROUP PORTIONS

FOOD GROUPS	PORTION SIZES
Grains	**Average calories per serving: 75 to 100**
Bread	
Sliced	1 oz. slice = 4" × 4" × ¼" thick
Pita	1 4" diameter, ½ 8" diameter
French or Italian	1 piece 2" long with 2" diameter
Rolls and buns	
English muffin	½ of 1" thick muffin
Burger roll	½ of a 2-piece bun
Bagel	½ 2" diameter

FOOD GROUPS	PORTION SIZES
Wraps	
Tortilla	1 7" flour or corn tortilla
Taco shell	2 6" cornmeal
Cereal	
Ready-to-eat	1 cup flakes or 1 single-serve box
Oatmeal, farina	½ cup cooked or 1 single unsweetened packet
Grits	½ cup cooked
Side-dish grains	
Pasta, any shape	½ cup cooked
Noodles	½ cup cooked (*not* instant noodle soups)
Rice, any color	½ cup cooked (*not* seasoned rice mixtures)
Couscous	½ cup cooked
Barley	½ cup cooked
Bulgur	½ cup cooked
Crackers	
Plain, square, low-fat types	8
Buttery, round types	6
Graham	3 squares or 6 of the smallest sections
Low-fat snacks	
Popcorn	4 cups air-popped or microwave-popped without butter
Pretzels	9 regular twists, 15 minitwists, 1 hard twist, 2 6" rods, or ½ 4" diameter soft pretzel twist
Rice or corn cakes	2 large round or 10 small round

Other grain-based foods that are made with lots of added fat and sugar do not belong in this group. Count them as extra-calorie choices.

Dairy and Substitutes	Average calories per serving: 100 to 125
Fat-free or skim milk	1 cup or 8 ounces
1% low-fat milk or skim plus	1 cup or 8 ounces

FOOD GROUPS	PORTION SIZES
Lactose-free, fat-free milk	1 cup or 8 ounces
Plain, fat-free, or low-fat yogurt	1 cup or 8 ounces
Flavored, fat-free, light yogurt	1 cup or 8 ounces
Cheese, hard, aged types	1 ounce or ¼ cup shredded
Cheese, processed, low-fat	2 ounces or 2 single slices
Cottage cheese, low-fat and calcium-fortified	½ cup
Parmesan cheese	4 tablespoons or ¼ cup
Soy milk, low-fat and fortified	1 cup or 8 ounces
Soy cheese, fortified	2 ounces or single slices

Frozen yogurt, ice cream, puddings, and other desserts made with milk are nonetheless desserts. They do not contain enough milk to nutritionally replace the dairy foods in your plan; they *do* contain a lot of other calories, especially from added sugar, so count these goodies as extras.

Meat and Substitutes	Average calories per serving: 75 to 100
Chicken breast, skinless	3 oz. or 3 thin slices or 1 boneless cutlet
Turkey breast, skinless	3 oz. or 3 thin slices
Chicken, dark meat, skinless	2 oz. or 2 thin slices
Turkey, dark meat, skinless	2 oz. or 2 thin slices
Fish fillet like cod, flounder, sole	3 ounces or 1 small fillet
Fish steak like salmon, tuna	2 ounces or 2" long × 1" wide × 1" thick piece
Shellfish (all types)	3 ounces = 9 large shrimp or scallops, ¾ cup clams, or ½ cup imitation shellfish
Game meats, buffalo, venison, ostrich, skinless duck breast	3 oz. or 3 thin slices

FOOD GROUPS	PORTION SIZES
Lunch meats	
<3 grams fat/oz.	3 oz. = 4 to 6 slices
3 to 4 grams fat/oz.	2 oz. = 3 to 5 slices
5 to 8 grams fat/oz.	1 oz. = 1 slice
Ground beef	
extra lean or 95% lean	2 oz. or ¼ cup cooked ground beef
85 to 75% lean	1 oz. or 2 tablespoons cooked ground meat
Beef steak or roast, well-trimmed	
Round, loin, flank	2 oz. or 2 thin slices
chuck, shoulder, brisket	1 oz. or 1 thin slice
Pork, loin chop, cutlet	2 oz. or 2 thin slices or ½ small boneless cutlet
Ham, fresh or cured	2 oz. or 2 thin slices
Lamb, roast or chop	1 oz. or 1 thin slice
Veal, roast or chop	1 oz. or 1 thin slice
Egg, whole large	1
Egg whites	3
Peanut butter, smooth or crunchy	1 level tablespoon
Nuts: peanuts, almonds, walnuts	2 tablespoons
Seeds: sesame, sunflower	2 tablespoons
Tofu	3 oz. or ½ cup
Veggie burger, fat free	2 oz.
Beans: navy, kidney, garbanzo	⅓ cup

All meats should be trimmed of any visible fat before and after cooking. When higher-fat-content cuts of meats are used, smaller portions must be eaten to stay within calorie guidelines. Processed meats like bologna, sausage, and liverwurst are typically 100 calories or more per ounce, so only low-fat versions should be used.

FOOD GROUPS	PORTION SIZES
Fruits	**Average calories per serving: 50 to 75**
Small oval: apricot, plum, kiwi	2
Medium round: apple, nectarine, orange, peach, pear, plum	1 = size of tennis ball
Large round: grapefruit, guava, mango, papaya, pomegranate	½
Berries: blue, black, raspberries	¾ cup whole
Strawberries	1 cup whole or 8 large
Grapes	20 small or 15 large
Cherries	15
Banana	6" long
Pineapple	½ cup cubes or 3 rings
Melon, cubed	1 cup
Cantaloupe or muskmelon	¼ of 5" diameter
Honeydew or casaba	⅛ of 7" diameter
Watermelon	1" thick slice
Avocado	¼
Raisins	2 tablespoons
Dates or figs, dried	2 whole
Mixed fruit, fresh or canned	¾ cup
Fruit juice, full strength	4 oz. = ½ cup

Heavily sweetened and processed fruits, such as the fruit fillings in pies and pastries, fruit spreads and preserves, and the fruit in yogurt do not count as a serving of fruit.

FOOD GROUPS	PORTION SIZES
Vegetables	**Average calories per serving: 50 to 75**
Artichoke	½ whole globe cooked or 4 hearts
Asparagus	1 cup cooked pieces or 10 spears
Beans, green or yellow	1 cup cooked pieces
Beets	1 cup cooked slices or 4 whole
Broccoli	1 cup pieces or 4 whole spears
Brussels sprouts	1 cup cooked or 8 whole
Cabbage, green or red	1 cup shredded cooked or 2 cups shredded raw
Carrots	1 cup cooked or 2 whole raw
Cauliflower	1 cup cooked pieces or 10 raw florets
Celery	2 cups diced cooked or 8 stalks raw
Chinese-style stir-fry	1 cup cooked
Coleslaw	½ cup including dressing
Corn	⅓ cup kernels cooked or ½ ear
Eggplant	2 cups cubed cooked
Greens, leafy	1 cup cooked or 2 cups raw
Lima beans	⅓ cup cooked
Mushrooms	1 cup cooked pieces or 2 cups raw or 14 whole
Okra	1 cup cooked pieces or 2 cups raw or 16 pods
Onions	¾ cup chopped cooked or ½ cup chopped raw
Peas, green	½ cup cooked
Peppers, sweet bell	1 cup chopped cooked or 1 whole raw
Potato, white	3 oz. whole
mashed	⅓ cup
Snow peas	1 cup cooked or 20 whole
Soybeans	⅓ cup cooked
Spinach	1 cup cooked or 2 cups raw
Squash, summer varieties	1½ cups cooked pieces or 2 cups raw
Squash, winter varieties	½ cup cooked
Succotash	⅓ cup

FOOD GROUPS	PORTION SIZES
Sweet potato	3 oz. whole
Tomatoes	1 cup diced cooked or 2 whole
Tomato juice	8 oz. or 1 cup
Vegetable juice	8 oz. or 1 cup

A serving of vegetables is more than a lettuce leaf and a tomato slice on a sandwich or garnishing a plate. Pickles and ketchup do not count as vegetables.

Fats	Average calories per serving: 50 to 75
Butter, stick	½ tablespoon
whipped	1 tablespoon
Margarine, stick	½ tablespoon
soft, tub-style	½ tablespoon
diet tub-style	1 tablespoon
Vegetable oil, all types	½ tablespoon
Mayonnaise	½ tablespoon
Salad dressing, vinaigrette	2 tablespoons
French or Dijon style	1 tablespoon
creamy styles	½ tablespoon
Tartar sauce	1 tablespoon
Cream cheese, block style	1 tablespoon or ½ oz.
soft, tub-style	1 tablespoon
whipped	1½ tablespoons
Sour cream	2 tablespoons
Light cream or half-and-half	2 tablespoons or 1 oz.
Gravy	2 tablespoons

Extras	Average calories per serving: 25 to 50

One rule: If you don't know the caloric value of something extra, don't eat it until you do.

☀ *MARISA:*

I had an almost all-carb diet—I'd just grab a bagel or a bag of chips or a candy bar and go. I rarely ate fruits and vegetables.

☀ *MARCHELLE:*

I quickly realized that if you can't figure out the ingredients in a particular meal, chances are it isn't too healthy. For example, I thought eggplant Parmesan was pretty healthy until I figured out it was 90 percent Parmesan and only 10 percent eggplant!

RESEARCH BULLETIN

Tufts University researchers found that the more often people of all ages ate in restaurants, the more body fat they had. Results showed they ate more calories and fat and less fiber than people who ate at home more often.

COPY THIS!

Table 2.6
PORTION SIZE COMPARISONS

Use these comparisons to estimate the weight or measurement of a food when it is of similar size to the items listed below. The items do not weigh what is suggested here.

FOOD PORTION	SIMILAR-SIZE ITEM
8 ounces meat	300-page paperback book
3 ounces meat	computer mouse, deck of cards, bar of soap, checkbook

FOOD PORTION	SIMILAR-SIZE ITEM
2 ounces meat	cassette tape, facial compact, stack of 10 small index cards, 3" × 3" × ¼" Post-it pad
1 ounce meat	3.5" computer disk, 1 CD, 4 stacked credit cards, 1 matchbook, 4 dice, 10 stacked business cards
1 cup	tight fist, baseball, tennis ball
½ cup	hockey puck, 3 square ice cubes, paper cupcake liner
⅓ cup	whole lemon, large egg
2 tablespoons	walnut in shell, golfball, Ping-Pong ball
1 tablespoon	thumb, wine cork, lipstick
1 teaspoon	thumb joint

RECOMMENDED READING

Dr. Shapiro's Picture Perfect Weight Loss: The Visual Program for Permanent Weight Loss (Rodale Press, 2000). Contains photographs of more than one hundred food portion comparisons.

3 ⅢⅢ➡

modern lessons in
label reading

PICTURE this: You walk down the frozen-food aisle of the grocery store and turn over every box of pizza in the freezer case looking for the one that has the fewest grams of fat per serving. When you find it, you buy it and later heat up a piece in the toaster oven back in the dorm. So far so good. Then, over the next hour, while trying to decipher your roommate's psychology lecture notes, you eventually eat all three pieces in the box. On the one hand, you feel relieved you found the lowest-fat pizza in the store. On the other, you are depressed that your raging appetite got the best of you again. But there's even more bad news.

A serving of *that* pizza is only one small section of the three that make up each piece—and *it* had only 3 grams of fat and 150 calories. But you just ate all 3 sections of all 3 pieces. By doing some simple math you quickly figure out that there were actually 9 servings in the box; therefore, you just ate 27 grams of fat and a whopping *1350 calories*. If this sounds familiar, you're not alone.

Most people are so focused on the metric numbers found on the nutrition facts panel—those grams of fat, protein, and carbohydrates and milligrams of sodium and cholesterol—that they overlook the most critical information found at the very top of the label: serving size and servings per container. These are *the* most important facts that will help you fight the freshman fifteen.

>※ *MARISA:*
I made the mistake of assuming the number of calories listed on the label was for the entire package and I had an expanded figure to show for it!

>※ *MARCHELLE:*
I often get a shock now when I look at the label of a small bag of chips and see that there are five servings in the bag!

One Size Does *Not* Fit All

Have you ever given any serious thought as to how you decide what serving is appropriate for each food you eat? Very likely your decisions are based on a mixture of how hungry you are, how much food is available, and how good the food tastes. Unfortunately, none of these criteria are hardwired to what your personal nutritional or caloric needs might be at any given moment. Sadder still is the fact that the food portions sold to us are getting bigger and bigger, so our frame of reference has become distorted.

If you have any doubt that food is morphing out of control, consider this: Soft drinks were originally sold in 8-ounce bottles. Convenience-store plastic cups now go up to 64 ounces. GULP! That is eight times more soda, and calories, than an entire gymnastics team needs to rehydrate.

It isn't just the food that is getting bigger, either. So are the cups and plates we eat with. Sets of glassware generally include three different sizes. The smallest glass, typically used as a juice glass, used to be about 5 ounces. Now the smallest glass in these sets is 10 ounces. A coffee cup traditionally held 6 ounces of hot java. In fact, that is the portion all coffee-making instructions are based on. Only problem is, coffee cups are now mugs that hold a minimum of 12 ounces each. The 12-ounce takeout cup is also the smallest one you can choose from the various sizes available at self-serve beverage counters.

In the not so distant past, standard dinner plates measured 9 inches in diameter. Today dinner plates are a minimum of 10 to 11 inches in diameter and, as you might expect, even bigger in restaurants. That spells real danger if you are a member of the clean-your-plate club, because the more room you have on that plate, the more food you can fit on it.

Even Mother Nature is doing us in. The fruit of yore would look meager compared to today's harvest. Apples and oranges actually *did* look like tennis balls a few seasons ago. Now round fruits are the size of softballs. Potatoes were generally 5 to a pound or $3\frac{1}{4}$ ounces apiece; we now get 2 potatoes per pound or a hefty 8-ounce spud when we skip the fries and go for a baked potato on the side.

There's no getting around it. If you don't know the portion sizes of what you are eating, you are eating too much. Read on to learn how to pay attention to what really counts on a food label when you're fighting the freshman fifteen.

Some Facts About the Nutrition Facts

◆ Serving sizes in the food plans outlined in chapter 2 and in most diet programs are different from the serving sizes on food labels—and very different from the amounts served in restaurants or normally prepared by people when cooking for themselves. But no matter where the food you are eating came from, it is essential to realize that your appetite does *not* dictate what counts as a serving.

✦ Government agencies decide what the reference amounts should be for different foods, and food companies must abide by them in declaring the serving size on a package label. Once you start scrutinizing those serving sizes, you will quickly recognize that the government is on a very tight food budget, as reflected in the minuscule portions they dish out.

✦ Serving sizes for similar foods are the same, so you can compare their nutrition information more easily. When looking at corn chips you'll see that the serving size is only 30 grams or 8 corn chips. Now even though no one ever eats just 8 chips, you can easily compare the fat content of different brands if you are so inclined.

✦ Serving sizes must be declared in both a household measure (cups, tablespoons) and a metric weight or volume (grams, milliliters). Some servings may also be declared as the number of "pieces" that make one serving based on the size or shape of the product, such as slices of cheese or squares of chocolate.

✦ Since all of the reference amounts are based on a metric weight, the household measure or number of units for similar foods may differ due to the different size or density of the products. For example, 30 grams is the reference amount for cookies. That may come out to only 1 Archway Fudge Bar, but 7 Nabisco Chocolate Snaps.

✦ The reference amount for soft drinks is 240 milliliters, or 8 ounces. Many beverages sold as single servings are actually in 12- to 24-ounce containers, which means you are drinking more than one serving and must adjust the caloric content given on the label to cover what you are actually getting if you drink the whole bottle or can.

✦ Serving sizes are based on the amount of the food as packaged. For many foods, like pasta, rice, and cake mixes, that serving size will change during cooking. Your only hope here is to know how much of the dry, uncooked stuff you prepared and what you added to it during the cooking, then decide what amount—one-half, one-third, or all—of the finished version you ate and base your calculations on that.

✦ Weight-control foods available only through weight-control programs may establish their own serving sizes for their products. Hence, the "diet" salad dressing with only 10 calories per serving looks really good compared with all the other brands with 25 to 100 calories per serving—until you pour the equivalent of 3 tablespoons on your salad and end up with 90 calories of dressing on 50 calories of lettuce. (Hint: The "diet" dressing used a serving size of 1 teaspoon while the other brands were based on 2 tablespoons, and there are 3 teaspoons per 1 tablespoon.)

✦ All of the nutrition information on a food label refers back to a single serving of that product as declared at the top of the panel. This means you simply must be able to do some quick multiplication in your head to figure out what you actually took in when you exceeded the recommended single serving.

✦ A nutrition facts label is not mandatory for all foods. If you've ever seen anyone carefully examining the hang tag on a pineapple or a head of cauliflower, it's probably due to the fact that nutrition labeling is voluntary on raw fruits and vegetables. If available at all, the nutrition facts for produce are found in brochures, display cards, or randomly attached tags.

✦ Voluntary labeling is also the case for foods in very small packages, like chewing gum and breath mints. These products are required to provide a telephone number or an address so that you can contact the manufacturer to get the nutrition information, if needed.

✦ Nutrient values reported on food labels are rounded up or down by as much as 10 percent, based on government regulations, since the actual content of a food can vary so much from farm to table. It is safe to assume that any underreported values are fairly evenly offset by the overreported ones, but just to be safe, round all your calculations up when keeping track of caloric intake.

✦ The % Daily Value information listed on the food label is based on a daily diet composed of 2000 calories, not necessarily *your* daily diet. It is not, therefore, necessary to try to reach 100 percent for each nutrient listed on the label if you do not need to eat 2000 calories per day. See Table 3.1 on page 38, **Daily Values for Different Calorie Levels,** to see what the goals are for your caloric level.

✦ Foods sold in restaurants, foods sold for immediate consumption (airlines, cafeterias), and foods prepared on-site (bakeries, delis) are exempt from nutrition labeling laws. Many restaurant franchises, however, do have the nutrition information for their menu items. They are supposed to be on posters or in brochures, but these are often out of date, out of stock, or no one working there has any idea where to locate them. To find the most current nutrition facts on the most popular franchise food chains, it is best to check their websites.

☼ *MARISA:*
After paying attention to serving size I realized how important it is to snack on healthy items like veggies and fruits, because they can fill you up and satisfy your munchies without all the calories of candy and chips.

Table 3.1

DAILY VALUES FOR DIFFERENT CALORIE LEVELS

Calories	Total Fat (g)	Saturated Fat (g)	Carbo-hydrates (mg)	Fiber (g)	Protein (g)
1200	40	16	195	20*	46**
1400	47	16	210	20*	46**
1600	53	17	240	20*	46**
1800	60	20	270	21	46**
2000	65	21	300	25	50
2200	73	24	330	25	55

* 20 g is the minimum amount of fiber recommended for all calorie levels below 2000.
** 46 g is the minimum amount of protein recommended for all calorie levels below 1800.
Cholesterol should be no more than 300 mg per day.
Sodium should be no more than 2400 mg per day.
There is no daily value for sugars in the diet.

First Impressions: Facing Off with a Food Package

Imagine you're dashing through the grocery store. You're in a rush, so you glance at all the yogurts in the refrigerator case and decide to grab the one that has the word *lite* in its name. Nice try, but that may not mean the same thing to the food industry as it does to you. Once again, you need to check the serving size and caloric content to see if what you're buying is *light* enough for you.

Believe it or not, a serving of cheesecake that has 200 calories and 4 grams of fat can be legally called "lite." That is because the regulations for a "light" or "lite" claim state that the product "must have ⅓ fewer calories or 50 percent less fat per reference amount." Since a reference amount of cheesecake has 300 calories and 8 grams of fat, the 200 calories/4 grams of fat version is, indeed, "lite."

It is also important to understand the semantics when it comes to the words *low* and *reduced* in a food claim. Check the three charts below for the basic definitions of each. Simply put, low is better. It generally means that the item has 40 calories or less, though there are several exceptions. But no matter what the exceptions, the "low" claim beats the "reduced" claim where it counts.

Here's why: All it takes to be called a reduced calorie/fat/cholesterol/sodium food is to come in with at least 25 percent less than the reference amount. The original food can be anything—pure lard or butter—but once you reduce the calories/fat/cholesterol/sodium by at least 25 percent, you've got yourself the "reduced" version. You have to read the rest of the nutrition facts to decide if it is reduced enough for you.

Also worth noting: Nutrition descriptions like "low" and "reduced" are *optional* on food labels. That means there may be items that meet the criteria but have not bothered to make that claim on the front of their package. Again, flip the product over to see what you get for the suggested serving size and whether that will fill you up without filling you out.

CALORIE CLAIMS

LABEL CLAIM	DEFINITION*
Calorie free	Less than 5 calories
Low calorie	40 calories or less**
Light or lite	⅓ fewer calories *or* 50% less fat; if more than half the calories are from fat, fat content must be reduced by 50% or more

* Per reference amount (standard serving size).
** Also per 50 g for products with small serving sizes. (Reference amount is 30 g *or* 2 tbsp. or less.)

FAT AND CHOLESTEROL CLAIMS

LABEL CLAIM	DEFINITION*
Fat free	Less than 0.5 grams fat
Low fat	3 grams or less fat**
Reduced fat	At least 25% less fat
Cholesterol free	Less than 2 mg cholesterol and 2 g or less saturated fat**
Low cholesterol	20 mg or less cholesterol and 2 g or less saturated fat**
Reduced cholesterol	At least 25% less cholesterol and 2 g or less saturated fat**

* Per reference amount (standard serving size). Some main-dish products and meal products, such as frozen entrées and dinners, have higher nutrient levels.
** Also per 50 g for products with small serving sizes (reference amount is 30 g or less *or* 2 tbsp. or less).

SODIUM CLAIMS

LABEL CLAIM	DEFINITION*
Sodium free	Less than 5 mg sodium
Very low sodium	35 mg or less sodium**
Low sodium	140 mg or less sodium**
Reduced sodium	At least 25% less sodium
Light in sodium	50% less sodium

* Per reference amount (standard serving size). Some dishes have higher nutrient levels for main-dish products and meal products, such as frozen entrées and dinners.
** Also per 50 g for products with small serving sizes (reference amount is 30 g or less *or* 2 tbsp. or less).

The Hidden Truth About Sugar

In their infinite wisdom, the feds have found a way to turn a really helpful consumer tool, the food label, into a shopper's worst nightmare when it comes to sugar content. Keep reading.

There are hundreds of foods in your grocery store right now that bear one of these claims on the front of the package:

- Sugar Free
- No Sugar
- Zero Sugar
- Without Sugar
- Sugarless
- Negligible Source of Sugar

yet they may list 25 grams of sugar or more on the nutrition facts panel on the side of the package. What gives here?

What gives is that the *claims* about sugar have to do with the sugary sweeteners that can be *added* to a food. Things like:

- Barley malt
- Brown sugar
- Cane sugar
- Confectioners' sugar
- Corn sweeteners
- Corn syrup
- Crystallized cane sugar
- Dextrin
- Dextrose
- Evaporated cane juice
- Fructose
- Fruit juice concentrate
- High-fructose corn syrup (HFCS)
- Honey
- Invert sugar
- Malt
- Maple syrup
- Molasses
- Raw sugar

- Rice syrup
- Turbinado sugar

to name a few. If none of these sugary ingredients have been added, then the manufacturer can make one of the above claims.

But if the food has a *naturally occurring* source of sugar, such as that found in any kind of fruit or grain or milk, the sugar from those ingredients must be included in the nutrition facts panel under Total Carbohydrate.

This explains, for example, why something as basic as a cup of fat-free milk has 14 grams of sugar listed on the nutrition facts panel, even though there are no sweeteners mentioned in the ingredients list. Milk contains lactose, lactose is a sugar, and the labeling regulations state that *all* sources of sugar must be included in the nutrition facts. Unsweetened raisin bran cereal also looks pretty sugary when you compare it with other cereals, but the sugar is contributed by the raisins, nothing more.

Making this already sticky situation even thicker than molasses are the sweeteners classified as "sugar alcohols." They are recognized by the "ol" ending in their names:

- Lactitol
- Maltitol
- Mannitol
- Sorbitol
- Xylitol

These ingredients add sweet flavors to foods, but are not technically classified as carbohydrates, so they do not have to be listed as sugars on the nutrition facts panel. Their use also allows manufacturers to place one of the "sugar-free" claims on the front of their package. But along with their perceived sweet taste, they provide about 4 calories per gram—just like sugar—and once again can get you into a lot of trouble if you aren't paying attention to the serving size and caloric content listed on the nutrition facts panel.

In fact, since so many people equate a claim like "sugar free" with "dieting"—and maybe you're one of them—the government has had to come up with a way to help people who might otherwise devour an entire box of so-called sugar-free cookies before they reach the checkout line. Here's what they've done. Any food that has one of the "sugar-free" claims and *does not* meet the requirements for a low- or a reduced-calorie food as described earlier in this chapter must declare that the product "is not a reduced-calorie food," or "is not a low-calorie food," or "is not for weight control," to protect consumers from an inevitable binge.

> ☼ *MARISA:*
> *I thought I was helping myself by eating low-fat and fat-free snacks I never realized how much more sugar those products contained.*
>
> ☼ *MARCHELLE:*
> *If you buy things in individual servings, it's way easier to keep track of how much you're eating. Just count the opened wrappers and containers!*

Weighing In with Artificial Sweeteners

When you wade through all the propaganda and scientific research about "intense sweeteners" (see list below), it's pretty easy to talk yourself into or out of either side of the debate. But here is what will matter most in the end: diversity.

What that means is this: You need to spread your options around when there is uncertainty about a new additive or ingredient in the food supply. If the substance has passed the first round of government approvals, it probably can't do you any immediate harm, unless you, as an individual, have an intolerance for the substance. Over a lifetime, you are exposed to many quite "natural" ingredients that may ultimately contribute to some disease later in life. We can never be sure of how much, or in what form, or in what combinations with other foods the risk is escalated.

UPDATE ON SWEETENERS

APPROVED INGREDIENT	BRAND NAME	SUBSTANCES UNDER REVIEW
acesulfame K	Sunett	alitame
aspartame	Equal, NutraSweet	cyclamate
saccharin	Sweet'n Low	neotame
sucralose	Splenda	stevia

Here's another point about "artificial" sweeteners to consider. What we do know about sugar and other "natural" sweeteners is that they contain calories, excess calories make us fat, and excess fat makes the body sick. If we want to eat or drink something that will taste sweet, we have to decide if we can afford the calories contributed by the sweetener used. If not, we can choose a lower-calorie alternative. If we do decide to use a substitute, we can switch around from among whatever is on the market so that we don't get too much of a questionable thing. Other than that, there's always good old H_2O, but in any case, when thirsty, be sure to read the label on those soft drinks before imbibing.

> ✳ *MARCHELLE:*
> *Some of those single-serving packages surprised me with the number of calories they contained. When I look at the serving size I try to ask myself if I can be satisfied with that amount.*
>
> ✳ *MARISA:*
> *When I was eating everything fat free, I would eat so much it would add up to more calories than if I had a regular serving of something that contained a little fat.*

Muscling Through the Meat Case

Processed meat and poultry items, such as packaged lunch meats and chicken franks, and all frozen entrées containing meat, poultry, or fish, are required to have nutrition labeling. Single-ingredient raw meat, poultry, and fish, like fresh ground beef, chicken breast, and rainbow trout, are not. They fall under a voluntary labeling program that states that the supermarket can make point-of-purchase materials available, such as brochures, posters, or signs, to provide nutrition information for these products.

The trick is remembering what you read if, in fact, the information can even be found. Then there is the problem of raw versus cooked-and-trimmed data.

The posted nutrition information for meat, poultry, and fish is based on the raw weight. Again, this is so you can compare the nutritional data on different cuts and types more readily. But meat shrinks during cooking as some of the moisture in it evaporates and some of the fat is melted. The edible portion becomes more dense and higher in protein and fat per ounce with the reduction in its water content after cooking. That, of course, will change the caloric content in a given serving, too.

Your best bet is to buy the cuts of meat and poultry with the lowest fat and caloric content in raw form and assume that it will still be true after cooking—as long as you are using a low-fat cooking method like broiling or grilling. It hardly matters what cut you buy if you're going to bread it and deep-fry it. You can also look for the packages that carry a "lean" or "extra-lean" claim as defined below.

MEAT CLAIMS

LABEL CLAIMS	DEFINITIONS
Lean	Meat, poultry, seafood, and game meat with less than 10 g total fat, less than 4 g saturated fat, less than 95 mg cholesterol per reference amount and 100 g.
Very lean	Meat, poultry, seafood, and game meat with less than 5 g total fat, less than 2 g saturated fat, and less than 95 mg cholesterol per reference amount and 100 g.

Meat by the Slice

The deli case can offer good sliced meat and cheese deals, but you need a friend behind the counter to find them. The only nutrition information available for the fresh sliced products being sold is what is on the label of the 5-pound blocks of meat and cheese displayed in the refrigerated cases. As that label gets peeled down during slicing, there may be little left to compare from one product to the next. The print on these labels is very small as well.

Asking the deli clerk for more information is worth the time and trouble. The biggest traps you must look out for are the many "low-sodium" meats and cheeses in the case—they are often still very high in fat and calories.

Presliced and packaged luncheon meats offer the greatest portion and calorie control. All the slices in a package are virtually the exact same size and the food label tells you how many calories are in each one, so all you have to do is count the calories when eating.

❋ MARCHELLE:
Eating shouldn't be like a chemistry class. I try to stick to foods that don't seem completely artificial.

❋ MARISA:
As a general rule, if you have no idea what is in the food you are eating, you probably shouldn't be eating it.

Natural, Organic, and Healthy—What Gives?

Instead of hassling with all this label reading and data analysis, wouldn't it be nice to be able to push your cart to the section of the store where the organic, natural, and healthy foods were all shelved so that you could just buy whatever was on sale there? Well, dream on, weary shoppers. There are no shortcuts through the food maze.

Still, there are those who cling to the belief that the fruits and vegetables they have handpicked from that segregated section of the produce aisle are, indeed, more wholesome than the mass-produced produce that surrounds it. Truth is, *all* of the food in your grocery store could be called natural, organic, and healthy—with the exception of pure mineral supplements like calcium and iron. Since they contain no carbon, they are not organic, but everything else that does contain carbon is, indeed, organic. You can confirm this in organic chemistry.

This is another case of semantics. First, there simply is no way to define the word *natural* and exclude any food we might seriously consider eating. Same goes for *healthy*. Any food can be eaten as part of a varied and balanced diet and be considered healthy, as long as it's not the only thing we're eating. More often, though, it's when we get too much of any one food that we run into the unhealthy problems.

The word *organic* is a bit different. While it literally means a substance containing carbon, there are laws that regulate the way food is grown and processed that allows them to be tagged as "organically grown" or "organically produced." This basically means that they have been made without synthetic fertilizers or pesticides.

There is no scientific evidence to support the notion that organically grown foods are healthier than conventionally grown ones. It appears plants don't know the difference between cow manure as a fertilizer and the white powdery stuff that comes in sterile 40-pound bags. What does affect the nutrient content of plants are things like soil conditions, climate, and handling during and after harvest.

A bigger concern facing all shoppers in the near future is the choice to use foods made from GMOs, or genetically modified organisms. This means that scientists have tinkered around with the DNA of the seeds so the plants will be more resistant to insects or grow faster or require less fertilizer. It also means there's more food to go around, at lower prices.

But what does all this tinkering mean for the future of your DNA? Good question, and one that maybe you will find an answer to if you're majoring in bioengineering. Otherwise, it's best not to lose sleep over things that you can't control when calories and portion sizes are in need of your constant attention.

4 ⅠⅠⅠⅡ➡

dorm-room
cooking essentials

ANY diet worth its calories is based on some type of food lists. You know, lists of foods you should eat, lists of foods you shouldn't eat, and lots of rules about how much, how often, and in what combinations. But these food lists are also the downfall of most diets, because in most cases the right foods are so hard to come by while the wrong foods are everywhere.

That is why we are telling you right up front that you have to take charge of your food inventory. You need to be the one deciding what foods will be in your pantry and refrigerator and to have complete information about the foods you select when eating out. It's your only hope of avoiding the hidden calories that lead to the freshman fifteen.

Inventory Control

The most rewarding thing about managing your own food supply is that you erase all those nagging doubts about how the food you're eating was prepared. Anyone who has ever tried to watch her diet has wondered about how much dressing was actually on the Caesar salad she ordered for lunch, or how much butter is coating the buffet vegetables, or if it was half-and-half or whole milk added to her coffee.

☀ *MARISA:*

My freshman year I really overindulged, like having two bagels for breakfast and a pint of Ben & Jerry's at night. I wasn't used to being surrounded by so much tempting food and didn't know how to limit myself. Once I started shopping for my food and fixing my own meals, I got my appetite under control again.

☀ *MARCHELLE:*

I once lived with three girls who had really poor eating habits. They would bake cookies every night and it was very tempting, but I found I could control myself if I drank a lot of water and satisfied my sweet tooth with frozen grapes and yogurt (see recipe for Creamy Frozen Fruit, page 171).

Keeping your own inventory of packaged and labeled foods and preparing easy meals for yourself allows you to always know exactly what you are eating. Observing the serving sizes on the labels and paying attention to the portions you take will let you know how much you're eating, too. By eliminating the gaps and guesswork about food, you will have the desire to stick to your program.

As with so many other things you're discovering in college, knowledge is power. Knowing as much as possible about the food you eat empowers you to make better food choices, which produces the results you want, which then reinforces the whole process for long-term success. As the rich and famous like to say, "Success breeds success." But the forever-fit crowd can chant that tune, too.

☀ *MARISA:*

A shopping list helps you focus on what you need and keeps you from wandering into the junk-food aisles. It also saves you money because without a list, you end up with a cart full of stuff that looked good but you really didn't need in the first place.

☀ *MARCHELLE:*

Grocery shopping is a lot like shopping for clothes. If I walk into a department store with no idea of what I'm looking for, I usually end up buying something I don't need and wasting a lot of time. Shopping with a list ensures that I will pick out the foods I need and get the job done quickly, which was always helpful with my busy college schedule.

The List

The first step to controlling what ends up on the shelves of your pantry and refrigerator is to strictly control what gets into your shopping cart. Yes, you must go grocery shopping and on a somewhat regular basis if you want to avoid the freshman fifteen. That is the only way you will have any hope of finding a fresh pear, a reduced-calorie bread, or sugar-free Popsicles in your dorm room.

Don't worry about how you're going to get to the market and lug all those shopping bags back to campus. You're not feeding a family of four and don't have a custom-built kitchen to work in, so the bags will be few and light. Chapter 5 provides answers to all your questions about where and how to get the food you need. Your attention right now should be focused on what you buy.

The simplest way to figure out what foods you need to buy is to check your shopping list. That's right, the one you've been jotting down things on all week so you'll know precisely what has to be replaced, refilled, or sought out when you get to the grocery store.

Calm down, this isn't as difficult as you may think. Part of the shopping list can be recycled every week. That's the part where you've itemized your "core staples." A list of the staples that complement the recipes found in chapter 11 is below. Once you modify this list of staples to suit your tastes and preferences, you can use it over and over again to replenish your personal inventory from week to week. It may help to keep it in a computer file for quick updating.

Keep your core list posted in a highly visible place at all times and just check off what gets used up during the week. Then all you have to do to complete your shopping list is add any perishable and "occasional" foods you may need. You may also find it convenient to help yourself to some of the items on your list that are readily available in the cafeteria, like packets of oatmeal, or to collect single-serving packets of condiments when eating out.

To be sure you have everything you need on your list and won't make any impulse purchases while roaming aimlessly around the store, check the weekly store circulars to see what's on sale or being featured with coupons and discounts. You can find out what fruits and vegetables are on sale, then add the best bargains from the produce aisle that week to your shopping list.

Next, check the dairy and deli ads for sales on the lower-fat products you regularly use so you can take advantage of their lower prices, too. Move on to see if any of your core foods can be purchased with a coupon or at a discount and note it on your shopping list. Now you can browse the seasonal and specialty promotions to see if there is anything new you want to try or substitute for a standard item on your list.

The trick here is that if you have done your homework and get the list right, you don't need to buy anything else and can save yourself a lot of time, money, and calories by avoiding anything that is not on it. For added restraint on your shopping impulses, be sure to shop with cash, and take only just enough, so that nothing superfluous lands in your cart.

✵ *MARISA:*
Coupons are a great idea if you have time to cut them out and the organizational skills to remember where you stashed them. If you're somebody who always balances your checkbook, you'll probably do fine keeping track of your coupons.

✵ *MARCHELLE:*
Club cards can save you a lot of money, too, and are easier to use. Just carry yours in your wallet or on a keychain and hand it to the cashier as you check out.

Core Staples

Pantry Items
Light bread: whole wheat, rye, seeded Italian,
    < 45 calories per slice
Low-fat tortillas: 6" to 8" diameter, < 100 calories each
Single boxes cold cereal: < 110 calories each
Single packets hot cereal: < 110 calories each
Low-fat microwave popcorn: 20 calories per cup,
    popped

Water-packed tuna: 3-ounce cans, 35 calories per ounce
Chunk white meat chicken in water: 98% fat free,
    35 calories per ounce
Canned vegetables: 8-ounce cans
    sliced mushrooms
    diced tomatoes or sliced stewed tomatoes
    chopped spinach
    quartered artichoke hearts
    chickpeas
    black beans
Canned fruit packed in unsweetened fruit juice or water:
4 ounces each
    pineapple chunks
    sliced peaches
    fruit cocktail
    applesauce
    mandarin oranges
Artificially sweetened ice tea and/or flavored beverage
    crystals
Dried fruit: raisins, cranberries, apricots, mixed fruit bits
Sliced almonds

Refrigerated Foods

Low- or reduced-fat cream cheese: soft or whipped,
    < 35 calories per tablespoon
Low- or reduced-fat cheese singles: < 40 calories per slice
Low-fat cottage cheese: < 90 calories per $^1/_2$ cup
Nonfat yogurt: plain or flavored and sweetened with
    aspartame, < 120 calories per cup
Eggs: large, or egg substitute: all egg or egg whites
Fat-free milk

Low-fat hummus and/or bean dip: < 25 calories per
  tablespoon
Low-fat packaged lunch meats: < 20 calories per slice
Light tofu: 8-ounce box

Condiments
Salsa (as hot as you like it): < 30 calories per ½ cup
Hot sauce: Tabasco or other brand
Low- or reduced-fat mayonnaise: < 50 calories per
  tablespoon
Single-serve packets:
  Ketchup
  Mustard
  Barbecue sauce
  Soy sauce
  Duck sauce
  Jam, jelly, marmalade
  Relish
  Horseradish
  Lemon juice
  Fat-free salad dressing
Nonstick cooking spray
Italian seasoning blend: oregano, basil, thyme
Cinnamon

Nonfood Items
Plastic storage bags
Paper towels
Dishwashing soap
Aluminum foil
Plastic wrap
Paper lunch bags

The Power of Packaging

Now that you're in the grocery store and have found your way to the cereal aisle and have even spotted your favorite brand, how do you decide which size to buy? The economy of unit pricing is not going to help here. Anything you buy cheap and in quantity can and will be eaten too quickly and casually, so avoid that trap and save yourself another few pounds. Instead, look for single-serving packages. In the case of cereal, you can really make your life easier by adding milk and eating right out of the miniboxes and plastic tubs.

Nothing beats the convenience of having your food in individually wrapped portions so you can just grab it and go without ever having to wonder how big a handful it was. You also don't have to deal with an opened box or container screaming out to you to take just one more or to finish it up so it doesn't go stale or get eaten by the other critters inhabiting your room.

When single servings are not available for items that are easy to eat in excess, be sure to have plenty of small plastic storage bags on hand so you can convert what you buy in bulk into preportioned quantities as soon as you get back to the

---

⛭ *MARISA:*

Portions matter! Don't eat anything by the handful. Get used to counting out the pieces using the recommended serving size on the package.

⛭ *MARCHELLE:*

Food is getting bigger and bigger. A simple muffin is now a megamuffin! Learn to cut big muffins and bagels in half and share them with someone or save half for the next day—just don't eat the whole thing all at once.

---

dorm. Make it a policy never to put away things like bags of pretzels or marshmallows or boxes of graham crackers or gingersnaps without first counting out the number of pieces that make up a serving and closing them up for rationed and rational consumption.

Picking Your Perishables

It's important not to buy more than you can eat of the foods that have a short shelf life for several important reasons:

- ✦ Overbuying leads to overeating
- ✦ Rotting fruit attracts bugs
- ✦ Wilting vegetables smell bad
- ✦ Spoiled meat is dangerous
- ✦ Wasted food deters you from buying more

If you want a variety of raw vegetables, it makes more sense to shop from the salad bar at the grocery store or campus cafeteria instead of buying whole heads of things you won't be able to finish before they turn brown. You also save yourself all the time and trouble involved when heads of broccoli or celery stalks have to be cleaned and trimmed.

The key to buying fresh fruits that you can enjoy eating for several days is to buy them in different stages of ripeness. There is no law against pulling apart the bananas to get the one or two you want off different bunches. Pick a yellow one for today and tomorrow, a greenish one for two days from now, and a greener one for the day after that. Do the same thing with other fruits that ripen after you get them home so there is always something ready to eat, but not all at once. Again, it is also handy to pick up an orange or some fresh fruit salad in the cafeteria.

Another way to avoid waste and overeating is by selecting the appropriate size when buying handheld fruits. That's right, even fruit has a proper serving size, and it's a $2\frac{1}{2}$-inch diameter, which is about the size of a tennis ball. Truth is, however, Mother Nature's bounty comes in many shapes and sizes, just like people, so you need to sort through the lot to find "average-size" pieces.

Fresh meat and poultry is typically sold in family-size packages that will need to be broken down for your dorm dinners. The butcher can be asked to repackage larger packages of chicken into 2-cutlet portions and pounds of ground turkey into quarter-pound packages, while the deli can just as easily slice and weigh your order into several 2-ounce portions instead of one 8-ounce package. Just ask.

To save yourself from the horror of pouring sour milk all over your cereal or, worse yet, taking a gulp only to spew it all over your sleeping roommate, be sure to check the last date of sale stamped on all your dairy products before purchasing them. Reach to the back of the refrigerated dairy case to find the cartons with the longest expiration time.

This is especially important because those dorm refrigerators do not maintain cold temperatures as well as full-size models. Every time you open that refrigerator door, warm air rushes in and raises the internal temperature for as much as an hour, depending on how much cold food you have stored in the unit. Buying half-pint cartons of milk from the cafeteria, or filling a takeout cup with just enough milk for one or two days, would be a practical solution to the spoiled-milk problem.

> ☀ *MARISA:*
> *I found that even if I didn't sit down in the cafeteria for a meal, I could use my meal card to shop for foods I could take back to the dorm to prepare and eat later. This sure saved me time, money, and calories.*
>
> ☀ *MARCHELLE:*
> *Once I figured which cafeteria had the best soup and salad bar and which one had the best stock of nonfat yogurt and fresh fruit, I made a point to go to that particular one when my supplies got low.*

Tools of the Trade

You've got your computer and cell phone to keep you organized and connected. Now you must make room for the other equipment that you need to sustain yourself. It's the kitchen stuff that will allow you to transform that fruit and yogurt into a frothy breakfast shake or those tortillas and salsa into a crunchy, spicy study snack.

Share the following list of equipment essentials with relatives and friends looking for the perfect high school graduation gift for you. If you're already on campus, prepare a wish list and E-mail it to the folks back home who might be worried about how you're "surviving" on your own. Tell them you discovered a few more "necessities" that would help make your life more bearable and then watch for the UPS delivery van.

Equipment Essentials

Appliances

- Refrigerator (the biggest one you can fit in, ideally with freezer space for more than a single ice cube tray and preferably self-defrosting)
- Microwave oven
- Electric hot plate
- Blender
- Toaster oven
- Electric hot water kettle
- Coffeemaker (optional)

Preparation Utensils

- Can opener
- Vegetable peeler
- 8" chef knife
- Paring knife
- Cutting board
- 8" skillet or frying pan
- 2-quart saucepan with lid
- Colander or mesh sieve
- Graduated set of measuring cups
- Graduated set of measuring spoons
- 16-ounce shaker jar with tight-fitting lid
- Flat spatula
- Large serving spoon
- Rubber spatula
- Ladle
- Baking sheet (to fit a toaster oven)
- Covered casserole dish (to fit a microwave or toaster oven)

Eating Utensils

- Dinner plates: 8" to 10" diameter
- Soup/cereal bowls: 16-ounce or 2-cup capacity
- Lunch plates: 4" to 6" diameter
- Coffee mugs: 8- to 12-ounce volume
- Small saucers/bowls: 8-ounce or 1-cup capacity
- Knives, forks, spoons
- Water bottle with retractable cap or built-in straw

Food Storage Containers

- Microwave-safe plastic bowls with fitted lids in small sizes and shapes
- Plastic storage bags in 2 sizes (for portioning food and storing opened containers)
- Clear, hard plastic bins with fitted lids (shoe box size) for spices and condiments

Cleaning Supplies

- Dishpan
- Sponges
- Dish detergent
- Wire soap pads
- Paper towels

Optional

- Disposable foil pans in different sizes
- Paper plates and cups
- Styrofoam cups and bowls
- Plastic knives, forks, spoons

> ✳ *MARISA:*
> *You must have measuring cups and spoons to be sure that what you are making will actually turn out the way it's supposed to. After all, there's a big difference between a tablespoon of Tabasco sauce and a teaspoon!*

MAKE NOTE OF KITCHEN MATH!

Table 4.1

LIQUID MEASURES AND EQUIVALENTS

1 gallon	= 4 quarts	= 8 pints	= 128 ounces			
1 quart	= 4 cups	= 2 pints	= 32 ounces			
1 pint	= ½ quart	= 2 cups	= 16 ounces			
1 cup	= 8 ounces	= ½ pint	= 16 tablespoons	= 240 milliliters		
2 tablespoon	= 1 ounce		= ⅛ cup			
1 tablespoon	= 3 teaspoons		= ¹⁄₁₆ cup	= 15 milliliters		
1 teaspoon	= 5 milliliters					

Measuring cups let us determine the volume of food we pack into the different-size cups, but they do not tell us how much that food weighs. Use Table 4.2 below to calculate the weight of a known volume of food. As noted in Table 4.1 above, there are 16 tablespoons in 1 cup, which can further help you calculate the weight of a smaller portion of any of these foods.

Table 4.2

DRY WEIGHTS AND EQUIVALENTS

1 cup of:	Weighs:
butter	8 ounces
flour	4 ounces

1 cup of:	Weighs:
sugar	8 ounces
milk	8 ounces
grated American cheese	4 ounces
grated Parmesan cheese	3 ounces
ice cream	5 ounces
ice milk	6.6 ounces
sherbet	6.6 ounces
flaked canned tuna	6 ounces
shelled nuts	3.5 ounces
peanut butter	9 ounces
cooked ground meat	6.4 ounces
cooked diced meat	10.6 ounces

Once you get into a routine of shopping for yourself, it will become a fairly simple task, like doing laundry on a regular basis. Just keep in mind that you are only cooking for one unless you have a roommate who would like to split the kitchen duties. There is no need to prepare more than you can eat at one meal or snack. Our recipes are so simple, you are better off making a fresh Chinese chicken salad for dinner than making a double batch at lunch and facing the possibility of eating it all before the dinner bell rings.

5 ⅢⅢ➡

finding food in
all the right places

ou can stop complaining about the cafeteria food, because we've heard it all before. By now even you should realize it's not where you buy your food or who's preparing it that can force you into avoiding skimpy spandex separates and into full-armor sweatsuits. It's the number of calories you're eating and the serving sizes, right?

So stop bad-mouthing the cafeteria food and check out what's worth eating in those havens for hungry guys and cheap chow. You might get more for your meal ticket than you ever bargained for! Then read on to find the places other than the cafeterias—within walking distance and within your budget—that can be used to get the food you need to stay in shape. Remember, we're talking shopping here, and if you can find the vintage clothing boutiques and bootleg CD vendors around campus, you can find food worth eating. It's just a matter of shopping like you mean it.

Dormitory Dining

The key concept here is making a distinction between Your Food versus Their Food. Consider their food anything your dorm mates are eating that you didn't put on your shopping list. If you have read and retained anything at all from chapter 4, you should realize by now how important it is to surround yourself with the kind of foods that will make *your* dorm pantry a figure-friendly place. It's *their* food, as in anything that is not yours, that can turn a mouthful into a mountain.

❉ *MARISA:*
The cafeteria was a dieter's nightmare for me. I found myself surrounded by a plethora of fattening, sugary, greasy, high-carb foods—and it was open until 2 A.M. so I could eat late at night.

❉ *MARCHELLE:*
Being away from home for the first time, the seemingly endless food on my meal plan changed my diet for the worse. Since the meal plan was already paid for, I ate a lot more than I normally would.

You are no longer in kindergarten where sharing was a golden rule. This is college, boot camp for the freshman fifteen, and you must abide by the platinum rule: Thou shall not share dorm food—ever. It's lifesaving decrees like this one that will also keep you from looking like the Michelin tire man when you don your skiwear on winter break.

Cafeteria Cuisine

Let's start with the obvious, the salad bar. If you time your visits to coincide with the freshest inventory, you'll be in produce paradise. You can make a salad to graze on while reviewing your notes for your next class, or assemble a platter of crunchy crudités to satisfy your appetite while studying later in the afternoon, or fill a takeout container with the fixings for some veggies you can microwave in the dorm with dinner.

As long as you are loading up on nude vegetables and fruits, you're fine. It's the non–garden variety items at the so-called salad bar that can get you into trouble, along with anything already dressed in fat. For example, bacon bits do not grow on trees. Neither do croutons and Jell-O. And while potatoes are a legitimate plant food, once buried under mayonnaise, as in potato salad, they are closer to being French fries than salad. See **Salad Bar Statistics,** on page 68, to help you get the most color and crunch for the fewest calories.

If the salad bar at your school looks like it's been on display too long, use the tongs to churn up the crisper foliage at the bottom of the serving containers. If they don't have an extensive enough assortment to meet your nutritional needs, complain to the head honcho. They do pay attention to requests for healthier foods, since it's good public relations to be known for the quality of your food.

☀ *MARCHELLE:*
Campus cafeterias usually have decent salad bars, but watch out for the fattening dressings and mayonnaise-covered mixtures. I learned to make my own dressings by combining different types of vinegar and lemon juice, then adding a little sugar substitute to cut the acidity.

If the dressings are all thick and creamy, you can dilute them with a spritz of vinegar or lemon juice to reduce their caloric content. If there are fat-free or lower-calorie choices available, you can also combine them with the high-octane ones to create your own calorie-conscious substitutes. No matter what dressing you end up with, however, be sure you use a spoon, not a ladle, to control how much gets added to your salad.

Salad Bar Statistics

15 calories per cup
Leafy greens, assorted types

5 to 25 calories per ¼ cup or 1 heaping serving spoonful
- Artichoke hearts, quartered
- Bean sprouts
- Beets, sliced
- Broccoli florets
- Cabbage, shredded
- Carrots, shredded
- Celery, diced
- Cherry tomatoes
- Cucumber, sliced
- Hearts of palm, sliced
- Mushrooms, sliced
- Onion, sliced
- Pea pods
- Pepper rings
- Radishes, sliced

25 to 50 calories per ¼ cup or 1 heaping serving spoonful
- Bean salad
- Cocktail corn
- Coleslaw
- Corn relish
- Pickled beets

More than 50 calories per ¼ cup or 1 heaping serving spoonful

	CALORIES
Olives	60
Potato salad	75
Chopped egg	75
Chickpeas	85
Pasta salad	85
Tuna salad	95
Imitation crab salad	95
Shredded cheese	100
Feta cheese	150
Bacon bits	170
Sunflower kernels	300

In addition to the salad bar, the cafeteria can also provide one-stop shopping for many things that are conveniently sold in single-serving packages. Scope out the selection of individually boxed breakfast cereals and instant hot-cereal packets on the breakfast bar to restock your pantry. Then grab some nonfat yogurt, half-pint cartons of fat-free milk, and string cheese from the refrigerated case.

Small cans, bottles, or boxes of full-strength juice can come in handy back in the dorm, along with mini cracker packets, whole fresh fruit, and hardboiled eggs still in their shells. If paper supplies are provided to wrap up takeout fare, help yourself to the sliced bread or pitas and sandwich meats at the deli counter and a whole baked potato from the hot-food line.

Be sure to check the soup du jour to see if it's something mostly made up of vegetables and legumes. If so, find a hot-drink container with a tight-fitting lid and fill it up so that you can reheat and sip that soup in the wee hours when everyone else is chanting "p-i-z-z-a."

The pasta station, taco bar, frozen yogurt machine, and bakery case are all very dangerous territory for the fledgling freshman fighting the infamous fifteen. Proceed past these cafeteria calorie traps with extreme caution at all times. If you do stop to indulge in one of these appetite suppressors, be sure to have all the figures worked out first. In other words, do you know how many calories are in a cup of cheese tortellini Alfredo? What's the diameter of those taco shells? Which yogurt topping has the fewest calories, strawberry or marshmallow? Can you eat just one-half of the fresh-baked oatmeal-raisin cookie now and save the other half for tomorrow?

If you can safely make it past those distractions, take a quick look at the hot-food lineup, or steam table, to see if there is any easily identifiable food being served there. Some aids to instant recognition would be the absence of gravies and sauces, no crispy crumb coatings, no baked-on crust or cheese topping, and no man-made shapes that are uniformly symmetrical—which is not the way Mother Nature makes things.

> ✭ *MARISA:*
> *Can you say candy? The weekly meetings at my sorority house featured every variety. I would eat it just because it was in front of me.*
>
> ✭ *MARCHELLE:*
> *There was a lot of overeating in my sorority house. Excessive amounts of sweets were always available.*

If you see something you can identify, like a baked chicken breast or a fish fillet, it is worth a second look. You see, you do need some kind of meat, fish, or poultry in your diet, or regular rations of their nonanimal counterparts like beans, soy, and nuts. Since these foods are not easy to whip up on the dorm hot plate, it helps if you can find something edible every once in a while in the cafeteria. The point is, don't disregard this area altogether. Give it a look and occasionally you might get lucky.

Sorority House Soiree

For those of you planning to pledge, we have some words of warning for all future sisters. Sorority houses are filled with every imaginable sweet treat you could ever want. Apparently, keeping a constant supply of these goodies on hand helps attendance at meetings. Be prepared to keep your hands out of the many candy dishes if you want to be able to wear those Greek letters with pride and no extra pounds.

Another caution for those who may end up living in a sisterhood house is the meal service. The refrigerator is always full and the food is homemade. Need we say more? Sitting around a table family-style means the gravy boat is going to pass by your plate several times before dinner is over. You'll need strong forearms (and fortitude) to keep it from making a stop on your potatoes with each pass.

After all is said and done, your decision to pledge or not to pledge won't come down to the quality of the food served at a sorority house, but it might give you a heads-up on what to look out for so that you can still fit into your spring formal after dining with the sisters for a semester. If, on the other hand, there's a Greek house with a fitness requirement and a gym on the premises, that might be the way to go.

> ✳ *MARISA:*
> *Think of the quickie mart as a one-stop shop for more junk food—too much temptation in too small a space.*

Campus Canteen and Neighborhood Quickie Mart

Think high prices and limited selection and you've got these places pegged. Of course, that will matter very little when they are the only food establishments open for business and you are starving. The one advantage about their merchandise is that most of it is packaged, which means the food has nutrition information on it to help you with the damage control needed at these desperate moments.

If you stick to familiar products with food labels, like canned tuna, boxed macaroni, and frozen vegetables, your only problem will be the dent in your food budget. No matter what, you should not enter the store until you have made up your mind what it is you are going in there to buy. Do not browse. I repeat, do not browse in places that specialize in temptation. You will surely find something that, for the moment, you believe you cannot live without for another second—but it's just not true. You will not only live without those 300 salty, greasy, sugary calories, but you will live far longer and happier without them.

If you're simply in a hurry and forced by a time shortage into shopping at one of these places, it might be more practical to buy one of the meal-replacement drinks or bars they stock and get out of the store as fast as you can. In fact, leaving any extra cash you may have on you in the car or back at the dorm will go a long way toward helping you to keep your wits about you when your stomach is growling.

Whatever the circumstances, avoid buying anything prepared on the premises and sold without a food label. There is no telling what's in those corn dogs or cheese nachos, but they're definitely high in calories. So are the jumbo "home-baked" cookies whose aroma is wafting out of the glass display case and the soft, doughy pretzels rotating in their own special oven. It may help if you think about all of the sanitation rules that were possibly broken by the hourly workers who handled those items before you arrived in the store. Yuck!

But you also need to watch out for the impulse purchases of hermetically sealed and packaged chips, ice cream, candy, and similar goodies piled around the checkout counter. They might satisfy you for the moment, but they will leave you disgruntled for days to come. And if you are going to go for the instant gratification, buy the smallest size available of whatever it is you're giving in to. Even earthquakes are measured, so if you're going to have one, let's hope it's low on the Richter scale.

FYI

Self-serve fountain drinks and dispensers of specialty coffees and teas are another source of innumerable calories. Whether you sip it or slurp it, if you swallow it you must count it. See chapter 6 for details.

☼ *MARCHELLE:*
The greasy burgers and fries at the fast-food chains were bad enough, but then we'd add a milk shake.

Fast-Food Fodder

Nothing can be all bad, right? So it is with fast-food franchises. They are conveniently located, offer quick service, and have familiar and consistent menus with moderate prices. But if you're interested in controlling the calories, fat, and/or sodium in what you eat, or increasing the whole grains, fiber, and produce in your diet, it's pretty slim pickings at these burger/taco/chicken joints.

Nonetheless, if you've gotta do it, then do it with a whole day of eating in mind, not just that meal. A carelessly ordered supersized burger, fries, and drink can cut a deep wedge into your daily caloric budget. The meal-deal dinner of three pieces of fried chicken with a biscuit and a shake can cut into tomorrow's calorie allowance. And a value-priced combo of a taco salad plus a burrito supreme could put you well into next week's account.

Your goal in these establishments is to find the lesser of the evils and eat only as much as you have to to hold you over until more suitable options are available. And the sooner the better. But once there, regardless of the sense of urgency you felt when you walked through the parking lot or pulled up to the drive-in window, it never makes sense to order more than you need because the price is better. There are many other ways to save money in life, but not as many ways to save yourself from spending calories on food you don't need that will turn into fat you don't want.

Some tips to help in that pursuit are to THINK:

◆ small, as in kids' menu, then get back to the dorm and eat a banana if you're still hungry.

◆ fussy, as in mix and match your own menu, don't take its "combo."

◆ snack, as in one item, like a single burger, not a meal, as in fries and dessert.

◆ healthy, as in salad or chicken that is grilled, not fried.

◆ smart, as in knowing the caloric value before you order, not after, when it's too late to change your mind.

◆ strategy, as in driving a little farther up the road to find a diner, where you'll have more choices.

All of the national chains have complete nutritional analyses for all of their products. You can access this information on their websites if the place you frequent doesn't have any of its product brochures on hand. Don't go into denial about this or make lame excuses or "only this once" exceptions. Find out what's in the food and make an informed decision about how, or if, you can fit it into your diet.

> ☼ *MARISA:*
> *Pizza, pizza, and more pizza pretty much sums up my freshman year. It was a social ritual late at night.*

Delivery Deals

College dormitories are like powerful magnets to pizzerias. Where there's one, you'll always find a half-dozen of the other. It almost seems as if they've got their ovens set up in the dorm basement so they can get their pies to your door before you change your mind. But this attraction is not just one of mercenary proprietors of pizza parlors preying on the endless wealth of college students' parents. Dorm dwellers are very attracted to pizza. In fact, if there were any value in recycled pizza boxes, there would be a fortune waiting to be claimed in the thousands of Dumpsters on college campuses all across America.

This propensity for pizza is like a computer virus that

spreads to everyone in your address book and immediately puts 5 pounds on each of them before he or she can download the shield. You see, nobody eats pizza alone. If someone four doors down missed dinner and orders a pie, everyone on the floor eats pizza. If your suitemate finds a roach in the bathtub, everyone on the floor eats pizza. If your new boyfriend shaves his head for the homecoming game and your parents are coming to campus to meet him, you and everyone on the floor eat pizza.

The surest solution to this epidemic is to develop a severe allergy to cheese. Obviously, you can't develop an authentic allergy at will, but with a really good imagination you can conjure up what it might feel like to have bloating and gas every time you eat cheese. Now try to imagine being bloated and gassy and 5 pounds heavier. You're sure to steer clear of a steady diet of pizza with that in mind.

Short of that, again you must be vigilant about how often and how much pizza is part of your college life. It is a communal food and college is a very communal experience, but so are the freshman fifteen! Take a look at these pointers before placing your order.

PIZZA POINTERS

Use these values for 1 slice of cheese pizza from a large round (18" diameter) pie cut into 8 slices, each slice having a 6" crust. If ordering from a national chain, check the website for nutrition information first.

PIZZA STYLE	CALORIES	FAT (G)
Thin and crispy crust	225	9
Hand-tossed	250	10
Thick crust	325	12
Stuffed crust	350	15
Sausage or pepperoni, add	50	4
Vegetable toppings, add	10	0

If there are other delivery services you can tap in to, start gathering up copies of their menus. You'll find them scattered about the mailroom, tacked up on bulletin boards, lying around in lounges and right under the door of your dorm room. If none of these sources produces results, check the phonebook or an on-line site for all of the nearby food-delivery services and call to get their menus faxed to you. Once you have a nice collection, follow these instructions.

1. Eat a sensible and satisfying dinner, then find a comfortable place to sit and take the menus, a phone, and a yellow highlighting marker.
2. Read each menu in its entirety—from appetizers to desserts—to identify anything that looks like it would be suitable for you to eat on your food plan.
3. Call the places whose menu descriptions are vague and ask questions to determine how dishes are prepared and what other ingredients are in them.
4. Highlight the items that have passed your screening test as being real foods that are not loaded with unnecessary calories.
5. Throw away the menus that do not offer anything you can/should eat.
6. Keep the marked-up menus in a folder near the phone where they won't get lost, because you are going to need them, and when you do, you will not be in a state of mind to do all the screening and scrutinizing you just did.

Takeout Time

The possibilities for takeout are limited only by your ability to carry the food that has been wrapped up for you. That's right, you are not confined to Chinese food and hero sandwiches. Any place that makes and sells prepared food can and will put it in a takeout container for you. Look at it this way: it saves them the trouble of pouring your water and cleaning up after you!

If you've patronized a local diner, sushi bar, or seafood restaurant with great food that didn't blow your calorie budget, use them again for takeout. Make a point of requesting a copy of the menu anywhere you dine off-campus that would be worth revisiting. These menus will come in very handy, especially on weekends when the cafeteria has closed, your refrigerator is empty, your stomach is growling, and your phone isn't ringing.

Rather than adding to your misery by eating the remains of a jar of peanut butter on an entire tube of raw cookie dough, you should call ahead to place your order for a nice meal. Then walk into town to get it and dine in your dorm by candlelight. Being able to dine alone, in style, is a skill you will no doubt need to use many times in life. Learn to do it now and you'll save yourself the unwanted pounds and uncountable calories eaten under duress.

✻ MARCHELLE:
I was thrilled to discover that most grocery stores have a sushi section—a big improvement for me over macaroni and cheese.

Grocery-to-Go

Besides your regular trips there for pantry staples and produce, the grocery store can be a great place to pick up ready-to-eat food without a lot of fuss. The best selections are in the "super" supermarkets, where you can even find tables for in-store dining. But most average-size stores will have a soup and salad bar, hot and cold delicatessen items, and some regional food specialties. Check out the features in the store nearest you and, once again, collect the menus where available.

Consider this: If you can buy a rotisserie-cooked turkey breast, a pound of grilled vegetables, and a half-pound of couscous, you will eat well for three days without once having to worry about whether the calories will fit.

Short-Order Cuisine

The best thing about diners, luncheonettes, and other counter-service eateries is that they can cook it the way you like it, because they cook to order. They are not dependent on pre-portioned, partially cooked, no-brainer foods that anyone passing through the kitchen could heat and serve.

Short-order menus give you the chance to customize your order. Say you're feeling a little anemic after a particularly heavy period and decide you need some red meat to replenish your depleted iron stores. You can go to a diner and order a lean, medium-rare, hot roast beef sandwich, but hold the bread, hold the gravy, and hold the mashed potatoes. In their place, you can have a side of stewed tomatoes for the vitamin C that will enhance iron absorption, and some sautéed mushrooms to flavor and moisten the meat. Ask for two slices of whole-wheat bread on the side so that you can make a sandwich with the surplus meat, then take it home to eat for lunch tomorrow.

In diners that offer breakfast, lunch, and dinner at any time of day (or night), you can view their menus as a big shopping list. Read each page to see what you need or want from each one (they tend to be lengthy), then compose your designer meal. For example, if you see spinach on the dinner side of the menu, you can request it in a two-egg-whites-one-yolk omelet for lunch. You can also ask to have a baked potato with some salsa on top instead of home fries with those eggs. Don't need the toast now? Then order raisin bread, untoasted, to wrap up and take back to the dorm to satisfy your sweet tooth later in the day.

BTW

The food served when you're sitting on a swivel stool in a bar is not the same as that which is served when you're sitting at the counter of a downtown diner. Don't even think about asking for low-fat dip with those buffalo wings at happy hour—it just won't happen.

Shopping-Mall Food Frenzy

The only reason to have so much food for sale at a shopping center is that the malls have gotten too big for the average, ablebodied shopper to cover in a single outing without sustenance. Oddly enough, the rations available could easily cause you to go up a size from what you were when you entered the mall if you stop too often for provisions. Then you're back where you started, standing in line to make exchanges!

A trip to the mall requires a well-planned strategy. If you have a tendency to impulse-shop, seek treatment, and fast. Because as sure as you're going to spend more money than you should satisfying that shopping impulse, you're also going to consume more calories than you should following the scent of cinnamon buns and sugar-glazed pretzels as you traipsc from one quadrant to the other in search of bargains.

The strategy you use should make it possible to shop immediately following a meal and make it safely back to the dorm with your purchases before another meal is needed. The worst thing you can do is arrive with an empty stomach and a full wallet. That's when $3.95 for a white chocolate mochaccino and another $1.95 for a chocolate-dipped biscotto—just to hold you over—can add up to 600 of your hard-earned calories.

Even things that sound sensible, like a fruit smoothie, a veggie wrap, and a chicken Caesar salad, can be caloric catastrophes when made in a food court. To avoid all temptation, try to stay in the main walkways of the mall, use the rest rooms located in the department stores, if needed, and keep a piece of chewing gum in your mouth until the shopping trip is over.

MARISA:
My freshman year I just ate whatever I was in the mood for regardless of calories or the size of the portion. I paid no attention to the healthier choices around me.

MARCHELLE:
I remember telling our mom I didn't want to go to college because I feared gaining weight like my sister did!

If you work in a mall and must eat there, make a point of getting to know the vendors in the food court and barter for bargains. The people behind those service counters are just working stiffs, too. Surely you can persuade a kind soul in the submarine-sandwich concession to make you a salad with some of that shredded lettuce, along with extra tomatoes and roasted peppers, then topped with sliced turkey breast or boiled ham. You can ask for a low-fat dressing from one of the burger giants and sanely proceed with your meal.

FOOD COURT FORAGING

	CALORIES	FAT (G)
FANCY-STYLE PRETZELS		
(One whole hand-shaped pretzel)		
Plain	340	1
Parmesan herb	400	10
Glazed raisin	470	1

Add calories and fat for the following		
Dipped in butter	40	3
Cheese sauce	100	8
Caramel dip	135	3

DELUXE COOKIES AND BARS		
(3 oz. or approximately 1 4" cookie or 6 minicookies)		
Chocolate chip	280	14
White chunks with macadamias	310	17
Oatmeal raisin	360	18
Fudge brownie	360	19
Coconut dream bar	400	25
Peanut butter	420	22

FRENCH-STYLE BAKERY		
(1 "standard" piece, ranging from 4 to 8 ounces)		
Plain croissant	250	6
Blueberry muffin	325	13
Lemon scone	370	8
Cheese danish	425	18
Almond croissant	570	38
Cinnamon sticky bun	675	35
Pecan bun	800	30

	CALORIES	FAT (G)
FROZEN YOGURT		
(Soft serve in medium cup or 6 fluid ounces)		
Nonfat and sugar-free	150	0
Nonfat vanilla	180	0
Low-fat vanilla	200	5

Add calories and fat for cones and toppings

Cake cone	15	0
Sugar cone	40	0
Waffle cone	110	1
Butterscotch syrup	130	2
Chocolate sprinkles	140	6
Hot fudge sauce	140	7
Wet walnuts	160	10

SUBMARINES AND HOAGIES

(6″ hoagie roll with dressing, lettuce, tomato, and onion)

Veggie and cheese	275	9
Turkey	300	10
Roast beef	350	13
Italian classic	450	30
Tuna salad	550	36

Add calories for mayonnaise, oil and vinegar, and cheese

Cheese, 1 slice	100	8
Mayonnaise, 1 schmear	100	10
Oil and vinegar, 2 tablespoons	100	10

SPECIALTY SANDWICHES

(Specialty sandwiches on 2 bread slices with spread)

Grilled chicken	450	20

	CALORIES	FAT (G)
Grilled cheese	500	30
Bacon, lettuce, and tomato	600	30
Egg salad	660	45
Corned beef Reuben	800	45
Turkey and bacon club	870	40

**Add calories for a side of potato chips,
potato salad, macaroni salad, or coleslaw**

MEXICAN STYLE

(One "standard" counter-service portion of each)

Chicken enchilada	350	20
Refried beans and rice	600	20
Cheese nachos	800	55
Beef chimichanga	800	46
Taco salad with everything	1000	70
(including shell for bowl)		

ORIENTAL STYLE

(Single-item entrées of approximately 1 cup)

Vegetable chow mein	200	8
Beef and broccoli	250	12
Sweet and sour pork	350	18
General Tso's chicken	350	15

(Side dishes of approximately 1 cup)

Steamed white rice	220	0
Chow mein noodles	250	15
Lo mein	270	10
Fried rice	400	20

Useful Websites for Caloric Content of Foods

- www.KenKuhl.com/fastfood
- www.dietitian.com
- www.nat.uiuc.edu
- www.nal.usda.gov/fnic/foodcomp/index.html

liquid calories— or how to get fat without even chewing

D RINKING your excess calories in the form of a beverage can produce the same amount of weight gain as chewing them in the form of solid food. In fact, it may do it a bit more surreptitiously because those liquid calories go down fast, without filling you up.

But a calorie is a calorie is a calorie no matter what food group it comes from, with the exception of the fermented and distilled category, also known as alcoholic drinks or beer and booze. These high-octane spirits can tip the scales upward in not one but *two* ways for anyone fighting the freshman fifteen.

"Proof" of Identification

Here's the first half of the drinking dilemma. Pure ethanol, or the alcoholic part of intoxicating drinks, supplies 7 calories per gram. The average drink has 10 to 15 grams of alcohol in it, or 70 to 105 calories from alcohol. Calories are also contributed by the other natural ingredients used in making wine, beer, and liqueurs. And, of course, calories are provided by whatever you mix those spirits with, like rum and *Coke,* vodka and *orange juice,* or Kahlúa and *cream.* (See **Mix-and-Match Alcoholic Beverage Calories** on page 89 for the details.)

The actual alcohol content in a distilled beverage can be determined by looking for the *proof* listed on the label for that product. The percentage of alcohol is one-half the declared proof. For example:

- 100-proof rum = 50% alcohol
- 80-proof whiskey = 40% alcohol
- 24-proof wine = 12% alcohol
- 12-proof beer = 6% alcohol

The fact that we have different standard serving sizes for the alcoholic drinks named above, such as 12-ounce bottles of beer and 1½-ounces shots of tequila, affects the caloric content of each drink as typically served.

ALCOHOLIC DRINK	STANDARD SERVING	CALORIES
Champagne, dry	5 ounces	85
Dry wine	5 ounces	100
Light beer	12 ounces	100
Liquor, 80 proof	1½ ounces*	100
Liquor,100 proof	1½ ounces*	125
Regular beer	12 ounces	150
Cordials, liqueurs	1½ ounces*	160
Ale	12 ounces	175
Wine cooler	12 ounces	200

* 1 ½ ounces is one measured shot.

The Double Whammy

The other way alcoholic beverages distort your figure, along with your equilibrium, is through the effects of intoxication. This is a purely sexist issue, but it's a very real one. You see, alcohol is carried in the body's fluids, which women have less of than men, not in the fat, which we have more of. Therefore, the same amount of alcohol is going to be more concentrated in the bloodstream of women's bodies than men's. Compounding the high is the fact that an enzyme that helps to mobilize alcohol and detoxify it through the liver is less active in women's bodies.

> ☀ *MARISA:*
> *The most popular drinks are the ones that are cheap and easy to make, like Jack and Coke or vodka and cranberry. As soon as you walked into a party, someone would hand you a drink.*
>
> ☀ *MARCHELLE:*
> *Beer is definitely the cheapest drink and the easiest one to serve at most venues.*

So while it takes all the willpower you can muster when you are cold sober to pass up the *free* stuffed potato skins and fried popcorn shrimp at the happy-hour buffet, you're doomed after just one drink. By then, your resolve is diminished and you'll be lucky if you can pass on the stale popcorn served at the bar.

Things just get worse after a second drink. That's when you might actually say right out loud to no one in particular, "I don't care how fat I get, I want to order some stuffed potato skins and I want them now!" Now the 300 calories of beer you have swallowed are being chased by 800 calories of grease and fat. But the damage doesn't end here.

At some point, you will have to go to the rest room, where you will inevitably catch a glimpse of yourself in the mirror under the worst possible lighting. Your hair and makeup are now askew from dancing, your eyes are red from the barroom smoke, and your vision is distorted enough to make you think you see an aura around yourself. It's not a pretty picture.

In that moment of horror you remember what you have eaten and decide to block the memory by having another drink—or two or three. By the time the evening is over, you have lost all discretion. You don't care how many calories are in *anything* or how bad you're going to look when all those extra calories show up on the scale as added pounds on Monday morning.

It is in this drunken and cavalier state of mind that you head out to the nearest quickie mart to buy a chocolate-covered ice cream sandwich and a box of crumb cake to comfort you through the rest of the night—neither of which you will remember having eaten come morning. Unfortunately, your body will.

Bottom line: Drinking and eating are almost as dangerous a combination as drinking and driving. Proceed with caution and be prepared to suffer severe penalties if you do not observe the calorie limits while under the influence.

MIX-AND-MATCH ALCOHOLIC BEVERAGE CALORIES

MIXER	AMOUNT	CALORIES
Club soda	any	0
Seltzer	any	0
Tomato juice	4 ounces	25
Bloody Mary mix	4 ounces	25
Orange, grapefruit juice	4 ounces	50
Pineapple juice	4 ounces	70
Cranberry juice	4 ounces	75
Ginger ale	8 ounces	80
Tonic	8 ounces	85
Regular cola	8 ounces	100
Regular lemon-lime soda	8 ounces	100

Just in case you end up at a party where they're whipping up some specialty drinks with exotic-sounding names and little umbrellas sticking up out of them, beware. These concoctions carry the triple threat of being:

- ◆ Bigger than your average drink
- ◆ Made with more total alcohol
- ◆ Delicious-tasting drinks that will go down easy

All of the above translate into more calories, quicker intoxication, and a bigger number on the scale in the morning.

☼ *MARCHELLE:*
In college, availability dictates what you drink, not what you want.

☼ *MARISA:*
I usually drank whatever was available. There was usually never any water in sight.

Even a more conventional mixed drink will make a higher caloric contribution to your evening than a single beer or glass of wine. Check out the calculations below:

MATHEMATHICS OF MIXED DRINKS

NAME OF DRINK	AMOUNT	CALORIES
Irish coffee	4 ounces	115
Tom Collins	8 ounces	125
Bloody Mary	8 ounces	185
Sangria	8 ounces	200
Manhattan	4 ounces	250

NAME OF DRINK	AMOUNT	CALORIES
Martini	4 ounces	250
Tequila sunrise	8 ounces	275
Piña colada	8 ounces	450
Daiquiri	8 ounces	450
Margarita	8 ounces	450
Mai-tai	8 ounces	600

TOP 10 REASONS TO STOP DRINKING

10. Drinking is against the law for people under age 21 in the United States.
9. "Beer belly" is not a myth.
8. A fellow student may be making a movie about college drinking for his film class and feature you in it.
7. The health benefits of red wine end after one glass.
6. Alcohol is a diuretic and toilets in bars are worse than those in the dingiest gas stations.
5. No one but professional flamenco dancers should try to dance on tables.
4. The food served in bars looks even worse coming up than it does going down.
3. You can get whiplash from doing shots too quickly.
2. Belching is not a guy magnet.
1. *Fighting the freshman fifteen!*

Liquid Calories Come in Many Flavors

One of the most significant public-health accomplishments of the twentieth century was the provision of safe drinking water in every American household. One of the biggest financial successes since the turn of the twenty-first century has been the sale of bottled water. There's no denying that Americans love their water and we want it in bottles bearing pristine designer labels. But that isn't all we're drinking these days.

The hot and cold beverage selection available for instant refreshment is bigger than ever imagined, and more options are being added every year. There are so many choices that a simple cup of coffee has become passé. Beverages are for sale everywhere we go and are being consumed no matter what we are doing. Cars even have beverage holders as *standard* equipment these days, as do some baby strollers!

It's time to take a closer look at all your favorite bevs to see what's really going down before you slurp yourself any closer to the freshman fifteen.

☀ *MARISA:*
I never drank soda until I went to college, but then, everybody drank it and I found myself drinking a lot more of it.

☀ *MARCHELLE:*
Girls seemed to like the fruit-based drinks and punches at parties over the beer and shots.

Coffee Concoctions

Not so very long ago, coffee was the drug of choice on college campuses. Many struggling freshmen had their first taste of the bitter grind the night before midterms and quickly learned that this legal stimulant was available 24/7. The stronger the brew, the quicker the buzz, so lighteners and sweeteners were clearly optional. Today you can add enough to a simple cup of coffee to turn it into a three-course meal.

Let's start with the blond option. Light cream or half-and-half are the standard coffee lighteners in better restaurants, diners, and popular coffee chains. They supply 30 calories per tablespoon or single little creamer container. Depending on how big that coffee container is and how light you like your brew and how many refills you get, the cream in your morning coffee alone can add up to 200 calories in no time at all.

In most places where cream is served there is also the option of getting whole milk, at a savings of 20 calories per tablespoon. Now this is something worth considering, and here's why: If you're currently using 6 tablespoons (about 1/3 cup) of half-and-half in that 24-ounce takeout in the morning, you could save 120 calories a day, or 840 per week, or an astounding 43,680 calories a year, by switching to whole milk. There's no denying that this would go a long way toward preventing the freshman fifteen. And we are only talking about that *first* cup of coffee of the day.

If you want to reap even bigger caloric savings, brew your own and lighten it with low-fat milk. Or you can go to a self-serve coffee counter, where you will find 2%, 1%, and fat-free milk, as well as lactose-free milk, fat-free internationally flavored creamers, nondairy creamers, and soy milk. Now we're talking *choice*. But in every case, you must remember, they lighten the coffee, not your figure.

COFFEE TIP:

Use nonfat powdered milk for your home brew and you'll get no fat, fewer calories, and lots of calcium from a milk product that doesn't go sour!

The next assault on that cup of coffee comes with the sweetener you choose. If it's sugar, you're adding 15 calories per teaspoon or single sugar packet. And it makes absolutely no difference if it's white, brown, or raw. If you use one of the artificial sweeteners, they average 4 calories per packet, mostly from the other powdery ingredients used to disperse them.

Now, if you don't think this little bit of sweetness is worth worrying about, try this: Hold on to *all* of your empty sugar or sweetener packets for a day to see how many you've used. Now multiply the number of packets by the calories per packet, then multiply it by 7 days a week, then by 52 weeks per year. Now what do you think?

✹ *MARCHELLE:*
Many of my friends and I indulged in drinks with lots of calories like soda and syrupy-sweet coffee drinks.

✹ *MARISA:*
We all drank the sugary, creamy coffee drinks like chocolate mocha and caramel latte, which are really high in calories.

CALORIES ON THE ROCKS

POPULAR BEVERAGE	AMOUNT (OUNCES)	CALORIES	FAT (GRAMS)
Dunkin' Donuts Orange Mango Fruit Coolatta	16	65	0
Starbucks Frappuccino	16	250	3
7-Eleven Früt Cooler orange cream	12	280	1
Friendly's raspberry sorbet smoothie	16	300	0
Ben & Jerry's Cappachillo Cooler with skim milk	22	320	0

POPULAR BEVERAGE	AMOUNT (OUNCES)	CALORIES	FAT (GRAMS)
McDonald's chocolate shake (small)	16	360	9
Häagen-Dazs Strawberry Sorbet Sipper	22	390	<1
Dunkin' Donuts Coffee Coolatta with Cream	16	400	19
Jamba Juice Kiwi-Berry Burner	24	470	<1
Dairy Queen Reese's Peanut Butter Cup Blizzard (small)	12	590	24
Dairy Queen chocolate malt (small)	15	650	16
Baskin-Robbins chocolate shake (large)	24	1,130	62

weekends, holidays, and visits home = dieting disaster zones

B E F O R E you've even had the chance to hold down a real full-time job with health-care coverage, a pension plan, and other company benefits, you get to experience in college what every member of the workforce likes most about their job: vacation time. That's because it is in college that you get your first exposure to one of the key characteristics of most jobs. They are filled with stressful deadlines and demands that leave you longing for an escape.

The weekends, semester breaks, and other legitimate excuses not to attend classes that occur at regular intervals as you pursue your degree can make up some of your most treasured memories of your college years. For one thing, they will give you something to look forward to in the midst of all that scholastic achievement day in and day out. And just as vacation time is meant to resuscitate a stifled worker, your collegiate time off will allow you to recharge your intellectual power cell for another stretch of higher learning.

Yet no matter how far you let your *mind* escape from the realities of your core curriculum as classes end each Friday afternoon or on the eve of an extended break, you cannot let your *body* escape with it. The vow you must be willing to make is that the body with which you start the weekend, vacation, or visit home is the one you will return with, for better or worse, till death do you part. Because just *one* new pound a weekend is all it takes to reach the predicated freshman fifteen by winter vacation.

The message here is this: It's okay to unwind, just don't unravel.

> ❄ *MARISA:*
> *My eating habits were just as bad over the weekends because the cafeterias were open as usual. . . .*
>
> ❄ *MARCHELLE:*
> *My weekends included a lot of late-night pizzas and movie watching.*

Weekend Warfare

A college semester is fifteen weeks long. That means your Monday-Wednesday-Friday lectures will convene forty-five times, you'll have to attend your Tuesday-Thursday labs thirty times, and there will be fifteen weekends for rest and recovery from it all. Those weekends are also notorious for extracurricular activities in which calories flow as freely as beer from a frathouse keg. In your efforts to combat the freshman fifteen, you must observe some weekend speed limits to be sure your Monday-morning weigh-in does not speed ahead on cruise control.

The first behind-the-wheel lesson to be mastered is that there are no "green light" days on the road to weight control.

This means that you should not delude yourself into believing that if you make heroic caloric sacrifices at every meal during the week, deny yourself so much as a taste of the foods you love from Monday through Friday, and perform Olympian acts in the gym night after night, you are entitled to eat nonstop from Saturday morning until Monday morning, when the red lights are all illuminated again. There is no such highway to travel.

Your best bet is to coast into the weekend with the amber light on, looking both ways before proceeding and keeping your foot near the brake pedal at all times. Calories are your constant travel companions and will cross your path at every turn. Be prepared to keep track of them all just like the odometer on a car records each mile it travels.

Another way to reroute your course around the hidden weekend speed traps is to start thinking about all the other things that make weekends fun besides the temporary pleasure of eating and drinking to excess. Food and alcoholic drinks are not the only draws at the party.

You can make it a point to consume all of the sights, sounds, and smells at every outrageous event you attend to refuel your starving senses after a week of tasteless brain food. And be sure to partake in the dancing, laughing, and cavorting going on all around you to revive your sedentary body after the numbing hours seated at computer terminals.

TWO IMPORTANT STATISTICS TO REMEMBER:

1. Studies have shown that restaurant meals contain 55% more calories than their home-cooked counterparts.
2. When eating out, 67% of Americans eat everything on their plates no matter how much is served to them.

A Crash Course in Motivation

A final itinerary to consider if you want a respite from toxic weekends and a tune-up for your weight-control engine is to schedule a "diet diversion" for Friday night through Monday morning. The purpose of a diet diversion is to give yourself a new focus for a few days so that you can return to your usual eating plan with renewed motivation. You can choose a theme for your meals, like eating only white foods for a day or following a "tonsillectomy" diet of soft liquids for another. Or you can just eat foods that begin with the letters that make up your initials. The point is, you'll be paying so much attention to the new rules of your diet diversion, you won't get distracted by the usual dieting decoys.

You can do anything you can think of that will steer you away from your customary approach to counting calories and controlling portions while offering you the challenge of something unfamiliar. It doesn't mean you are not responsible for calories and portions while on this detour; you'll just have a new way of looking at them for a few days. This may be all you need to stay the course until that alarm clock goes off on Monday morning when you can once again work toward your dieting destination with renewed resolve.

Look over these diet diversions to get ideas for your alternate routes.

DIET DIVERSION 1: WHITE FOOD ONLY

The calories and portions must still be in compliance with your food plan, just keep the selections colorless.

Breakfast   Vanilla yogurt, cream of wheat, and canned pears.

Lunch   Egg-white omelet filled with onions and potatoes and a (peeled) cucumber salad.

Snack   Saltines with jack cheese and a quartered apple (peeled, of course).

Dinner   Broiled flounder over white rice with cauliflower and snow-white
               mushrooms.

Treat   Angel food cake with low-fat whipped topping and a glass of milk.

DIET DIVERSION 2: SOFT-LIQUID PLAN

Eat only those foods that don't require rigorous chewing—think tonsillectomy or
wisdom-tooth extraction.

10:00 A.M.   Monkey Shake (see recipe, page 173).

12:00 P.M.   Tomato and tofu soup.

2:00 P.M.   Jar of baby food peaches.

4:00 P.M.   Soy Fruit Pudding (see recipe, page 174).

6:00 P.M.   Pureed lentil and carrot stew.

8:00 P.M.   Frozen fruit bar.

10:00 P.M.   Hot cocoa made with fat-free or soy milk.

DIET DIVERSION 3: EAT YOUR INITIALS

Limit your choices to foods that start with the same letters as your name, as in
the example for **M**arisa and **M**archelle **B**radanini.

	M FOODS	B FOODS
Fruits:	mango, melon	banana, berries
Dairy:	milk, mozzarella, and muenster cheese	buttermilk, Brie, and blue cheese
Vegetables:	mushrooms, mung beans, mustard greens	bean sprouts, beets, broccoli, baked beans, Brussels sprouts
Meat:	meat loaf, meatballs, macadamia nuts	bologna, brisket, bass, bacon, Brazil nuts
Grains:	muffin, macaroni, melba toast, matzoh	bagel, bread, bran flakes, barley, bulgur
Fat:	margarine, mayonnaise	butter
Treats:	M&M's, Miller Lite	brownie, Bud Light

> ✸ *MARISA:*
>
> *I always ate better on vacation with my parents because we would go out to nice restaurants, where I could order fish or sushi. Weekend trips with friends were filled with junk food and drinks.*
>
> ✸ *MARCHELLE:*
>
> *If I went home for the weekend my meals were more complete because my mother was preparing them. She would make dishes I never had the time or know-how to make.*

Holiday Rehabilitation

Semester breaks generally coincide with major holidays and the end of a major segment of the academic year. This means you have no doubt just finished a week of late nights spent cramming for exams and frantically trying to finish whatever projects were still due to avoid the dreaded "credit deferred" for incomplete work. You probably didn't get as much exercise as you should have and very likely ate more calories than your food plan called for.

But once you're on your way to the resort or to the slopes or to visit a roommate's hometown, your alibi for careless eating and insufficient activity ends. Cramming may have helped get you through finals, but it's definitely not a successful dieting strategy. So if you're still skipping workouts, eating endless carbs, and losing count of your calories by noon each day, you're also getting perilously close to the freshman fifteen.

The fact that you don't have to sit through boring lectures all day does not mean you get to celebrate by eating from dawn to dusk. Not even close. It does mean you'll get to sleep a bit longer, relax for the better part of your day, and certainly have more fun than you do when attending classes.

One of the splurges you should try to squeeze into your vacation budget is plenty of recreation. Scout out things to do that you can't or don't get to do on campus. The physical activity will be a welcome change from all the mental activity of your course load, and it won't hurt your weight-control efforts, either.

If you're headed for someplace dominated by sun, sand, and surf, sign up for one or more of the following events to "recreate" yourself while away:

Recreation à la Sol

Beach volleyball	Acrobatics	Whitewater rafting
Water aerobics	Trampoline	Water polo
Windsurfing	Cricket	Unicycling
Kayaking	Tango lessons	Scuba diving
Surfing	Snorkeling	Water skiing
Sailing	Canoeing	Paddleboating

If your travels take you to sweater and earmuff territory, you can count on your appetite climbing as your body temperature drops. But you can't rely on shivering alone to burn off all the calories you may consume in the form of wassail, cheese fondue, and hot apple cobbler à la mode as you try to thaw your inner being.

A frigid climate demands vigorous activity to stoke the internal furnace while separating you from the generous warmth and caloric abundance of the kitchen stove. Then as you engage in these polar sports, you can burn enough calories to earn a place before the hearth and enjoy the hearty fare being served there.

Sign up soon for one or more of these frosty outings to melt fat cells no matter what the temperature is outside.

Fitness in the Frigid Zone

Curling	Ice fishing	Spelunking
Hiking	Ice hockey	Ice sailing
Ice skating	Luge	Cross-country skiing
Orienteering	Rock climbing	Downhill skiing
Sledding	Snowshoeing	Tobogganing

✸ MARISA:
There were a lot of weekend trips where everyone piled onto a bus and our only stops were at fast-food restaurants.

✸ MARCHELLE:
On most group trips there was a disgusting amount of beer and bad food around.

One Price Does Not Fit All

If you and your buddies landed a great deal on an all-inclusive trip to some resort, or anywhere where the words *all-inclusive* actually include all the food you can eat at the nonstop buffet and all the alcoholic beverages you can drink from the twelve strategically located bars, you will definitely need a new dictionary to redefine what *all-inclusive* means for you.

First, get over the idea that you have to eat and drink your share since you or your parents have already paid for it. The packaged price you pay for airfare, ground transportation, hotel, meals, and "beverages" is already saving you, or your parents, plenty, regardless of how much you eat and drink. The law of averages also has you covered in that your modest level of consumption is needed to offset the behemoth intake of some other bottomless pit who booked the same rate as you.

When you do make your first expedition into the round-the-clock international self-service smorgasbord, be prepared to follow these crucial steps to ensure that you will not have any expanded areas of flesh to cover with sunscreen by the time you finish eating.

☀ *MARISA:*

There was always plenty of free alcohol available on trips. What kind of food we had didn't seem to matter.

Step-by-Step Guide Through the All-You-Can-Eat Buffet

1. Wear something fitted at each meal—preferably a swimsuit if allowed.

2. Try to avoid eating at the peak times where the crowds are hungry and rude and the fight for food can lead to combative choices.

3. Do not take a tray or plate upon entering the food arena. Keep your hands clasped together and your eyes wide open.

4. Examine every serving station to take note of what is available and worth eating. Make special note of homemade breads, rolls, and croissants and all the dessert options so that you can budget for them, if necessary.

5. Decide how many of your allotted calories you can afford to spend for that particular meal, knowing that others will follow or have come before.

6. Use only the midsize to small plates to gather your food as a method of volume control. Make-believe you are fixing a plate for a child or that you are a food critic on assignment and in need of only a tasting portion.

7. If you must take a full-size dinner plate, do not let any of the food you put on it touch one another.

8. Select your food in courses—appetizer, salad, soup, entrée, dessert—so that you must return to the lines if you really want something else.

9. Utilize scrupulous portion control to enjoy a taste of some of the higher-caloric offerings. Don't waste calories on foods that taste the same no matter where you get them, like black olives or American cheese.

10. Skip anything you can get anytime unless you're relying on it as an appetite suppressant, like oatmeal with raisins or a baked potato with marinara sauce and Parmesan cheese.

11. Leave uneaten on your plate anything that actually looked a whole lot better than it tasted—especially in the dessert category. Why eat a dessert that doesn't taste great?

12. Signal the waitstaff to clear your plate if you are returning to the food arena for something else so there's no incentive to pick at what's still on it.

13. Check the time when you finish your meal and decide when you can reasonably expect to be hungry or need to eat again. Don't get caught up in eating on other people's schedules just to keep them company.

Making Your Way Back Home

If you've been eating sanely up to this point, there's no need to stuff yourself with Mom's cooking while you're at home. You must do everything in your power to discourage your family from treating you like a contestant on a *Survivor* show who hasn't eaten in six weeks. You need allies on the home front, so let them know what you are really looking forward to—

sleeping in your own bed, hooking up with old friends, and shopping with your parents' credit cards.

✺ MARISA:
At college I had easy access to virtually every kind of junk food, so that's what I found myself eating. No one came to my dorm room at 6 P.M. and told me it was time for dinner like Mom did when I was at home.

✺ MARCHELLE:
During the holidays I liked having a little bit of all those fun holiday foods—but I learned not to stack my plate three feet high!

If you fail to convince them and return home to cupboards full of your prepubescent fixations, like Twizzlers red licorice and Drake's coffee cakes, and dinner menus featuring crescent rolls, penne with vodka sauce, and pecan pie, you need to level with them. Tell them you are auditioning for a spot on the college debate team and a requirement is that you must fit into one of the existing blazers. A similar case can be made for a part in a campus play, orchestra, or other activity where costumes or uniforms are needed.

The same holds true for those care packages and travel coolers they're so willing to send back to campus with you. This type of hospitality is as lethal as a book of gift certificates to Dairy Queen. The necessary antidote is an E-mail to Mom before you arrive home listing all of the groceries you would like her to buy for you so that you can make it through the final weeks of the semester without reaching the freshman fifteen.

Familial Food Traits

Just as your red hair and short fingers mark you as a member of a certain genetic lineage, your eating habits have been passed on, too. While they may not be coded into your DNA, there is much about the way you eat that is shared with your family of origin after years of repeated exposure and behavioral conditioning.

This evolutionary link usually weakens when someone (that's you) moves away from the nuclear family and adopts eating habits compatible with a new age and environment. Trouble is, the folks back home have not branched off onto the new food chain with you. So when you do return and take your usual seat at the family table, you must be careful that you don't also slide back into your adolescent diet. It probably wasn't the most nutritionally sound or calorically balanced when you were fourteen, and it surely isn't what you want to be eating now.

For instance, you may have adored French toast with strawberry jam and powdered sugar for a special breakfast when you were growing up. If your mom or some other well-meaning relative offers to make it, be sure those are the calories you want to start your day with. If not, tactfully tell her or him what you would prefer instead or agree to make your own breakfast when you get up. This might be a good time to introduce your siblings to the Creamy Melon Bowl (see recipe, page 159) or the Burrito to Go (see recipe, page 159) you've grown to love while away at school.

Your family may also want to take you out for dinner to your once favorite Australian steak-house restaurant with the fried onion chrysanthemum appetizer and chocolate decadence dessert that you adored eating after winning a field hockey game in high school. When the subject comes up, that may be a good time to tell them about your newfound fondness for the sweet-and-sour cucumbers and curried rice of Thai cuisine, and that you know of a great new Thai restaurant nearby.

If your relatives are the kind of people who like to use food to show you how much they've missed you—as in preparing too much of it and endlessly offering you more—it is your job to fill them in on all the other things you *really* want them to do for you during your short visit home. Mention things that utilize their talents and make them feel needed, like sewing a patch on your favorite jeans, or finding your old Buffy the Vampire Slayer costume in the attic for campus fright night, or balancing your checkbook for the last three months. That should keep them out of the kitchen for a while, anyway!

Care Packages That Count

We can now get food absolutely everywhere we go, even when there is no good reason to be eating, like while filling our car with gas. Yet with all this limitless food service, there is still a strong urge among parents to send food to their college students. Apparently these parents think their child is bright enough that they're willing to make a one-hundred-thousand-dollar investment in her education. They believe she can register for her classes, buy her own books and supplies, remember to brush and floss her teeth, and occasionally change the sheets on her bed, but they do not think that she will be able to find the cafeteria or a grocery store on her own.

The sooner you set some boundaries on this goodwill giving, the less likely it will be that your parents will have to pay for your sessions with a weight-loss counselor when you return home for the summer. Use the food lists in chapter 4 to specify exactly what it is you would like your family to purchase for you. Better yet, if you've been doing your own grocery shopping up to this point, don't relinquish control over your pantry now. Ask for gift certificates to the store you normally use back at school or request use of Mom and Dad's debit card so that you can do your own shopping while at home.

> ☀ *MARCHELLE:*
> *Some of my friends got these ridiculously enormous care packages—sometimes on a weekly basis—filled with cookies and other sweet treats. They would earn points with the R.A. by placing some of their stuff on a plate at the entrance to the dorm so that we could all eat it.*
>
> ☀ *MARISA:*
> *Most of my friends received care packages loaded with home-baked goodies. My care packages were full of healthy treats once my family saw how much weight I was gaining.*

If sending you back to campus empty-handed is going to be too much for the folks to bear, give them a list of *nonfood* items they can supply. That way your food budget will go further because you won't be using it to pay your phone bill or keep your clothes clean.

NONFOOD CARE PACKAGES

HAIR CARE	SKIN CARE	DENTAL CARE	CLOTHING CARE
Shampoo	Facial cleanser	Toothbrush	Laundry detergent
Conditioner	Toner	Toothpaste	Stain remover
Gel or mousse	Moisturizer	Dental floss	Dryer sheets
Hair spray	Complexion cream	Mouthwash	Bleach

KITCHEN CARE	**AIR CARE**	**BODY CARE**	**FOOT CARE**
Dish detergent	Room freshener	Bar soap	Sweat socks
Sponges	Scented candles	Shower gel	Shower sandals
Paper plates	Incense	Bath powder	Shoelaces
Paper towels	Odor-Eaters	Deodorant	Slippers

APPLIANCE CARE	**COMMUNICATION CARE**	**CLEANING CARE**	**DECOR CARE**
Copier toner	Postage stamps	Disinfectant	Duct tape
Print cartridges	Calling cards	Window cleaner	Poster tacks
Computer paper	Stationery	Carpet cleaner	Lightbulbs
Batteries	Cellular service	Furniture polish	Picture hooks
	GCs*		

ENTERTAINMENT CARE

Compact disks

Videos or DVDs

Movie theater GCs

Magazines or novels

* Gift certificates

ALSO WORTH CHECKING OUT:

Handheld calculators and computer software programs that track your calories, fat, and fiber intake, and more, plus analyze what food groups you have eaten from.

boredom, stress, and pms—the triple threat to weight control

As if you didn't have enough opportunities to overeat while away at school, the triple threat of boredom, stress, and PMS can definitely push you closer to the freshman fifteen if you don't learn how to diagnose and treat them from the very minute you arrive on campus. It is important to remember this: Food is *not* a curative for any of them. Read on to find the right remedy for what ails you before gaining weight becomes a chronic condition, too.

Dying of Boredom

Though no one has actually ever died of boredom, the condition does exist, and for many it has surely kept them from dying of starvation. The site of the affliction is the mind or, more accurately, the imagination, of the sufferer. For some college students, in spite of all the course work, sporting events, partygoing, gossiping, club participation, wardrobe decisions, Internet browsing, excuse-making, party hunting, and career planning, boredom does occasionally strike.

> ✴ *MARISA:*
>
> *I was most bored during some of my three-hour lecture classes. I resorted to snacking to stay awake—and, unfortunately, it wasn't on fruits and veggies.*
>
> ✴ *MARCHELLE:*
>
> *I stayed pretty busy my freshman year with campus activities and joining a sorority, but late afternoons were pretty relaxed. I was most vulnerable to boredom grazing then.*

The telltale signs of boredom are captured in these common complaints:

- "I don't have anything to do."
- "I have so much to do but don't feel like doing it right now."
- "There's nothing to do around here."
- "I wish I had something to do."
- "This place is so lame, there's never anything to do."
- "Does anybody want to do something?"
- "Is there anything going on anywhere?"

When you encounter these symptoms of boredom, it is vital that you isolate yourself from the sufferer because her condition will quickly advance to the more contagious stage of the disease, eating for a cure. That is when you will hear remedies such as these:

- "Who wants to order some mozzarella sticks and marinara sauce?"
- "Does anybody feel like going out for a cappuccino and some gelato?"
- "I'm in the mood for tacos, anyone want to join me?"

"Let's bake some cinnamon buns with this biscuit dough."

"How about we all go into town to the Old Country Buffet?"

"What happened to all that candy left over from the Halloween party?"

Eating is very stimulating, so it does seem like a quick cure for boredom, but eating for entertainment only makes the condition worse. That is because when you have finished the first "dose" of eating, you will still be bored, plus you'll feel lousy for eating so much.

Thinking about the food you'd like to eat, then *figuring out* how to get it and *enjoying* the taste and texture of it once you do are all behaviors that can be redirected to eradicate boredom without your gaining an ounce. The treatment requires that once you or your friends are bored, you need to think about something you would like to do, decide when, where, and how you are going to do it, then go have a good time doing it. Food need not play a role in your recovery from boredom at all, unless, of course, you happen to be bored at the same time you are hungry, in which case you may end up planning your next meal.

10 Time-Honored Treatments for Boredom

1. Wear your swimsuit under some sweatpants, jog to the fitness center, dive in the pool, and swim laps.
2. Place your favorite dance music CD in the player, turn up the volume, then get everybody on the floor into the halls and start dancing.
3. Type up all your course notes for your history class.
4. Get a deck of cards and find someone to play gin rummy with.

5. Read all the editorials in the school newspaper, then write an op-ed comment.
6. Find at least two other people and a long piece of rope and go outside to jump rope—double Dutch.
7. Read and outline an entire chapter for one of tomorrow's classes.
8. Write a long, newsy letter to a grandparent.
9. Load your camera with film and walk around campus photographing all your favorite spots.
10. Do your laundry.

> ⚙ *MARISA:*
> *When I was stressed, I ate whatever was within grabbing distance, usually a bag of chips and a candy bar.*
>
> ⚙ *MARCHELLE:*
> *My first encounter with college-level test taking was by far my most stressful period as a freshman. That's when I turned to caffeine.*

Stress Test 101

In many ways, being stressed is the exact opposite of being bored. For college students, it starts the very first moment you pass through the campus security gates on move-in day—a classic time for stressful flare-ups in the life of a college freshman. You can hear the tension in your parents' voices as they jostle for a parking space within a quarter-mile of the dorm so they can help you unload the car of all your worldly possessions. Only then do you discover the elevators are slow or nonexistent, and your footlocker full of sweaters feels like it's full of sand.

By the time you reach your room, your roommate has already taken the best bed, mattress, and desk. Then as you unpack your clothes and try to fit them into the too small closet and the too few bureau drawers, your stress level grows more intense. Be prepared for these additional aggravating conditions:

- ◆ Finding enough outlets for all of yours and your roommate's electronic devices
- ◆ Making space for her musical instrument and your artwork portfolio
- ◆ Having the wrong room keys
- ◆ Getting a serviceperson to hook up your prepaid phone lines
- ◆ Tracking down a maintenance worker to turn off the heat blasting into your room on this August afternoon

The goal for the next four years, and for the rest of your life thereafter, is not to seek food as a sedative to relieve your stress. Deal with whatever is bugging you, or deal with eating, just don't do both at the same time.

RESEARCH BULLETIN:

Women who eat while doing something else eat 13% more than women who are not distracted while eating.

Deconstructing Stress

What you are actually experiencing when you get "stressed out" is a perception about your situation and circumstances that leaves you feeling helpless and overwhelmed. Someone else in the same situation may be quite calm and in control.

You, on the other hand, may fare much better under the pressure of final exams and term-paper deadlines than some of your roommates.

The fact remains that stress is first and foremost a perception, not a clinical condition that affects all people in the same way, like strep throat. This means you have a far greater chance of controlling whether or not you're going to get stressed out over the hair clogging the bathroom sink than you do of catching the athlete's foot being shared in the shower stalls.

The hormones produced in the body in response to this perceived stress will also add to your misery. That is because they stimulate your appetite *and* fat storage—a deadly combination if ever there was a way to be done in by your own hormones!

Your best antidote to stress is to defuse whatever it is that's triggering it, even if you just forget about it for an hour or two until you can compose yourself. Think of it as a "de-stressing" time-out. Go sit in a quiet corner and clear your head of all negative thoughts for a while. And if you feel any urge to eat, you must first ask yourself the question "Am I really hungry?" If the answer isn't a resounding, unequivocal "Yes!" then delay eating, too.

It's all a matter of adjusting the way you look at your circumstances and improving your coping skills. A certain amount of perceived stress is both normal and necessary in a balanced life, but there is no need to be in a constant state of unrelenting stress. When that is the case, other physical problems usually show up as a result of the way the stress has been internalized.

The lack of sleep, lack of exercise, and poor eating that accompany a stressful existence weaken the immune system and leave you more susceptible to infection and other opportunistic illnesses. Then when you become physically sick while still stressed out, your chances of perceiving your situation in a more favorable light fall even lower and your condition worsens.

Even if you do not get pushed beyond your stress tolerance by the demands of college life, you will still be exposed to some annoying, unavoidable stressors. And just as with boredom, trying to get relief by eating is not a cure. If you have any doubts, take a close look at the numbers next to the list of **Stress Escalators** below. To suppress these stressful appetite stimulants legally, and with no unpleasant side effects, use any of the methods in the **Stress Reducing Checklist**.

☀ *MARISA:*

I would eat anything with lots of sugar in it to help me stay awake when I had to write papers or study for exams. I would skip meals, then eat anything to get me through the endless studying.

Table 8.1
STRESS ESCALATORS

	Amount	Calories	Fat
Candy			
Butterscotch	1 oz. / 5 pieces	115	1 g
Candy corn	¼ cup	180	1 g
Caramels	5 squares	170	3 g
Chocolate chips	¼ cup	335	21 g
Chocolate-covered peanuts	10 pieces	210	13 g
Chocolate-covered raisins	10 pieces	40	1.5 g
Fudge	½ ounce	60	1.5 g

	Amount	Calories	Fat
Gumdrops	10 small	135	0
Jelly beans	10 large	100	<1 g
Lollipop	1 small	25	0
Marshmallows, miniature	½ cup	100	0
Milk chocolate	1 ounce	145	9 g
Peanut brittle	1 ounce	130	6 g
Peanut butter cups	1 cup	135	8 g
Praline	1 ounce	130	7 g
Taffy	1 ounce / 2 pieces	120	1 g
Toffee	1 ounce / 2 pieces	130	8 g
Truffles	1 ounce	130	9 g

Cakes

	Amount	Calories	Fat
Brownie	2" square	140	7 g
Carrot cake	1" slice in 2 layers	240	11 g
with cream cheese frosting	1" slice in 2 layers	485	30 g
Cheesecake	1" slice	450	35 g
Chocolate cake with frosting	1" slice with 2 layers	450	15 g
Coffee cake with crumb topping	2" square	240	12 g
Cupcake with icing	1	175	6 g
Lemon pudding cake	2" square	245	10 g
Pound cake	½" slice from loaf	230	9 g

Cookies

	Amount	Calories	Fat
Animal crackers	10 pieces	115	3.5 g
Butter cookie	1 2" diameter	25	1 g
Chocolate chip cookie	1 2" diameter	55	2.5 g
Creme-filled sandwich	1 cookie	50	2 g
Gingersnaps	4 / 1 ounce	120	3 g

	Amount	Calories	Fat
Marshmallow with chocolate coating	1 cookie	60	2.5 g
Peanut butter sandwich	1 cookie	65	3 g
Oatmeal raisin	1 2" diameter	55	2.5 g
Shortbread	1 2" diameter	65	4 g
Sugar cookie	1 2" diameter	60	3 g
Sugar wafers with creme filling	1 bar	20	<1 g
Vanilla wafers	1 small	25	1 g

OPEN IN CASE OF EMERGENCY!

Stress-Reducing Checklist

❏ Go to the gym to soak in the hot tub, then turn on the jets to revive yourself in the whirlpool.

❏ Turn out all the lights and meditate by candlelight.

❏ Plug in the aromatherapy machine and breathe deeply.

❏ Heat up a warming pad and apply alternately to your forehead and to your abdomen.

❏ Practice holding different tai chi positions for 3 minutes each.

❏ Borrow a vibrating cushion and place it under your bare feet while you massage your temples.

❏ Drop your chin to your chest and slowly rotate your neck from right to left, holding for a count of 5 on each side. Repeat 5 times.

❏ Watch a stand-up comedian on the Comedy Channel and laugh out loud.

❏ Go to a playground and ride the swings.

❏ Slowly raise your shoulders to your ears while inhaling through your nose, hold for a count of 5, then slowly lower your shoulders while exhaling through your mouth. Repeat 5 times.

❏ Sit in a chair in a sunny spot in the periodicals room at the library and read all the comic strips in the daily newspapers on file.

☀ *MARCHELLE:*
I definitely craved chocolate when I had PMS. I found if I tried to abstain, I ended up overindulging, so I allowed myself to have small amounts to regulate my cravings.

☀ *MARISA:*
I did not have PMS, but some of my friends did. Soup, 7 Up, and saltine crackers were staples for them at that time of month.

PMS and LBS

Up to 75 percent of menstruating women complain of one or more symptoms of premenstrual syndrome (PMS) each month. These complaints include:

Mood swings	Crying spells	Breast tenderness
Depression	Headache	Bloating
Anxiety	Fatigue	Swelling
Irritability	Cramping	Lower backache
Anger	Cravings	Overall aches and pains

If you are familiar with any of these symptoms, they are not in your head.

Most of the 150 reported symptoms associated with PMS are believed to be due to the hormonal fluctuations that occur throughout the menstrual cycle. The changing levels of hormones such as estrogen and progesterone are responsible for many of the physical changes in the body, like swelling and cramps. These physical changes, in turn, are believed to trigger some of the mood swings experienced. This is compounded by shifts in other hormones, like serotonin and norepinephrine, which directly impact one's emotional outlook.

Here is just one explanation of why you can go from being happy and self-confident one minute to feeling tearful and pathetic the next.

Ovulation begins approximately fourteen days after the onset of the last period and is marked by an increased production in the hormone progesterone. Higher levels of circulating progesterone slow the rate in which food moves through the digestive tract.

The longer food remains in the intestines, the more water the body can absorb from it. If the diet has also been higher than normal in sodium during this critical time, the kidneys will respond by holding on to more fluids to help dilute the excessive sodium in the cells.

In a few days the combined effect of this water retention can result in 2 to 5 pounds of added weight that can lead to the swollen ankles and fingers, bloated abdomen, tender breasts, and tension headaches many women experience. That alone is enough to make anyone depressed, angry, or irritable.

The slower transit time also allows colonic bacteria more exposure to the undigested waste material passing through the final five feet of the large intestine. This extended bacterial fermentation can produce cramps, flatulence, constipation, and diarrhea. Being irregular will affect anyone's disposition, but when combined with muscle tension, backaches, and joint pain, it isn't hard to understand why personalities deteriorate during this time of the month.

The only premenstrual symptom that is not as easy to explain is the craving for sweets or, more specifically, chocolate and salty snacks. These specific cravings are not widely seen or consistently experienced by women around the world, suggesting they may be more culturally than biologically influenced.

But for women in the United States, these cravings are very common. One reason may be that little girls in this country begin to worry about their weight while still in elementary school and they begin dieting while only at single-digit ages. This constant sense of deprivation and obsession over food makes it very easy to seek gratification from the most tempting but typically forbidden foods when feeling out of sorts—as you do when you're premenstrual.

It's as if the body has its own logic, which argues, "It's not fair we have to do without the foods we love when everybody else gets to enjoy them!" So in defiance many women reach out for their beloved comfort foods at that point each month when they most need a little extra comfort. This, of course, can have dire effects on weight control.

Since there are nine months in an academic year, that's nine menstrual cycles for the average freshman woman, plus the empathy eating that goes on when anyone living with her or in close proximity to her is having her period. That's a lot of potential PMS pounds contributing to the freshman fifteen. Fortunately, there is a way around this vicious cycle.

The best defense against the monthly distractions of PMS is a consistent daily approach to diet, exercise, sleep, and stress management. And isn't that what this whole book has been about so far, anyway?

Regular meals made up of plenty of fresh fruits and vegetables with adequate amounts of whole grains and lean proteins will keep your body in better balance as the premenstrual time approaches. These are the foods that supply the needed vitamins and minerals to offset water retention and keep the bowels emptying efficiently. These fresh, less processed foods are also lower in added salt and help to keep sodium intake under control as well.

Getting enough aerobic exercise provides a means of eliminating excess fluid via perspiration and helps to raise the level of some feel-good hormones, the endorphins. Making sure you are getting sufficient rest reduces feelings of fatigue and irritability.

While there is no cure for PMS other than menopause, you can minimize the symptoms that can lead to added weight. But you can't wait until the cramps and cravings begin. You have to eat, exercise, and sleep right all month long to be physically prepared for the hormonal changes brought on by your menstrual cycle. Then the changes your body undergoes will be less extreme and your emotional response will be more manageable. One great way to "manage" those cravings is to reach for one of the satisfying suggestions that follow.

Curbing the Cravings

Crunchy Creations

Spicy Macho Nachos: see recipe, page 168.

Ranch Veggie Mixer: see recipe, page 167.

Squirrel Mix: Combine any or all of the following: seasoned fat-free croutons, Chex, Cheerios, Cheez-Its, sesame sticks, soy nuts, popcorn, and pretzel nuggets. Scoop into a paper cup and nibble away.

Spoonable Morning Glory Muffin: Combine ⅓ cup fat-free granola with ½ cup applesauce or pineapple tidbits, 1 grated carrot, 1 tablespoon raisins, and/or 1 tablespoon chopped nuts.

Sweet Addictions

Fiber 'N Fruit: see recipe, page 169.

Banana Boat: see recipe, page 175.

Almost Apple Pie: Toast a slice of raisin bread and top it with low-fat cream cheese and apple butter.

Banana Cream Oatmeal: Prepare 1 packet of instant oatmeal and stir in a mashed banana and vanilla yogurt.

Easy Fruit Sorbet: Place 1 cup of small pieces of your favorite canned fruit in a plastic storage bag and freeze. (Pears, peaches, apricots, and fruit cocktail work best.) Microwave the bag for 10 seconds to soften slightly, then empty the fruit into a blender container and puree.

Dutch-Chocolate Oatmeal: Combine 1 packet of instant oatmeal and 1 packet of nonfat sugar-free hot cocoa with 1 cup of boiling water, then sprinkle cinnamon on top.

Instant Mocha Pudding: Combine 2 tablespoons of sugar-free, fat-free instant chocolate pudding (save the rest for another time) with ½ cup skim milk and 1 teaspoon instant coffee granules in a shaker container with a tight-fitting lid. Shake vigorously for 2 minutes until partially thickened, then chill for 5 minutes to thicken further.

Spicy Sensations

Chicken Teriyaki Sammie: see recipe, page 163.

Mini Chicken Burrito: see recipe, page 164.

1-2-3 Pizzas: (1) Season tomato sauce (or ketchup, if desperate) with garlic powder, basil, and oregano. (2) Spoon sauce over saltine crackers. (3) Sprinkle with Parmesan cheese.

No-Fat Nachos: Dip white-cheddar popcorn cakes into 3-alarm salsa.

Chinese Pretzels: Dip pretzel sticks in the hot Chinese mustard left over from takeout.

Curried Tater: Top a baked (or microwaved) potato with fat-free sour cream or plain yogurt and a generous dusting of curry powder.

Mini Cocktail Shrimp: Buy a single shrimp cocktail in a jar and place 1 shrimp at a time on an oyster cracker.

Winter Wassail: Heat up apple juice with cinnamon, nutmeg, and/or cloves and dunk with gingersnaps.

> ❉ *MARCHELLE:*
>
> *My roommate and I did end up on the same cycle. We found it easier to control our cravings if we shopped for fruits and veggies a few days before. Also, there's nothing like a hot bath to make a girl feel better.*

Useful Websites

Keep in mind, girls, no matter how bad a day you may be having, you never have to go it alone. A kind word and a friendly message are as close at hand as your keyboard. Check out these websites for useful guidance and support during "that time of the month," or at any time at all.

For self-directed meditation lessons: www.wildmind.org

For women's health issues: www.4women.gov

For weight-loss counselors and chat rooms: www.Cyberdiet.
com—free

www.eDiets.com—about $10 / month

www.Nutrio.com—about $10 / month

www.ABCweightloss.net—$20 to join

www.DietSmart.com—$45 to start

guys and
other saboteurs

T HERE are two virtues you cannot rely on when you are trying to control your weight: willpower and won't power. This
means that no matter how strong you think your willpower is
to adhere to your daily caloric allowance, you *will* pig out on
graham crackers smeared with cake frosting after you find out
your lab partner lost all the data you collected for the first biol-
ogy experiment. It also means that no matter how great your
conviction is to go to the gym four times a week, you *won't* be
willing to get up early to go before your morning class after
blowing it off in the afternoon to watch your boyfriend play
flag football.

The lesson here is that you are going to stray from the path
and other people are going to help you do it. The sooner you
face that fact, the quicker you'll recover from the lapses and
resume your fight against the freshman fifteen.

No one can make you feel inferior without your consent.

—Eleanor Roosevelt

> ✺ *MARCHELLE:*
> *There is really a big transition when you leave home and move into the dorm. There is a lot of pressure to eat and drink all the time.*
>
> ✺ *MARISA:*
> *I wish I had remembered the advice to only eat when you are hungry. I was always eating and snacking as a social thing.*

Facing Your Foibles

The most important question you're going to have to answer this semester is this: "Who are you controlling your weight for?" If the answer you come up with is anyone's name other than your own, you are headed for a failing grade. Here's the real deal.

There are many things about ourselves that we *cannot* change. Most of our physical features are genetically predetermined and strongly influenced by the social and temporal environment in which we were raised. No chance of changing any of that now that you're in college. Much of our personality is also hardwired, then fine-tuned by the nurturing we received early in life. Little hope of unraveling any of those connections, either.

Yet for some bizarre reason, the vast majority of us go through life believing we can change ourselves to conform to what other people think we should look and act like. This makes no sense whatsoever and is a tremendous waste of our allotted time here on earth.

Once you acknowledge this bit of truth, you can get to work on those aspects of your makeup that are amenable to change, namely your behavior and your attitude. Each of us is empowered with the ability to control how we behave and how we feel about and react to the things that happen to us, but not necessarily how we look.

You can start by accepting your body exactly as it is and letting that feeling of unconditional love for the body you now have govern how you take care of it from here on out. You'll be astonished by all of the time and energy you'll have then to devote to changing other behaviors, if you care to. That means you can get excited about making your own Tropical Sunrise Shake (page 174) every morning for breakfast or counting the number of laps you run around the track because you're not constantly bummed out about having thick ankles or bony knees.

Once you feel good about yourself in your present size and shape, there's little chance you're going to get too upset if other people tell you otherwise. They may be entitled to an opinion, but that doesn't mean they're right. But we also know what can happen when we feel bad about our bodies and someone reminds us of our flaws. We attack the thing we despise by filling it with more and more food. Then we really have something to feel disgusted about and the cycle continues.

The moral: Love your body and see who wants to join you. Now, with that said, let's see how we can get this message across to the guys.

> Be yourself. Who else is better qualified?
>
> —Frank J. Giblin II

Leveling the Playing Field

It's a given that women's bodies have been objectified through the ages, in every culture and by every medium, starting with men's eyes. And yet, no matter how hip we are to the changing "ideals" set before us by the fashion and entertainment industries, we continue to strive for their illusive perfection. Don't you think it's about time to stop the never-ending makeover?

The first step toward freedom from the tyranny of the male gaze is to disarm men of their power over your identity. If women no longer allow men, or anyone else, to determine how they're going to feel about themselves, the unwelcome remarks will fall on deaf ears and begin to sound like gibberish.

Then you can launch the counterattack and hit them with a blast of their own medicine. For every unwelcome remark about your shape or appearance, you must have an arsenal of rebuttals ready to fire back. You can go after their obvious imperfections or simply set the record straight on whose opinion matters most. Either way, you are undermining their assumed right to tell you how you should or shouldn't look. And once they are over that, we might all be able to get along a whole lot better. Check out this artillery to find your weapons of choice.

When he comments on your appearance: *"If I don't look good to you, maybe you should have your eyes checked."*

When he turns to look at another woman: *"You may think she looks hot, but she's definitely cool on you."*

When he makes suggestions about your size: *". . . and those jeans you're wearing would sure look better if they were 32/34s."*

When he says you need to tone up: *"I'm fit enough to exercise my option to walk out on you."*

When he compares your body/appearance to a celebrity's or supermodel's: *"Let's remember, if I looked like that, I certainly wouldn't be here with you."*

> ✷ *MARISA:*
>
> *I saw plenty of girls who tried to impress guys by drinking way more than they could handle, which always ended up bad.*
>
> ✷ *MARCHELLE:*
>
> *I think the meal plans are too big for most people. You find yourself eating more just so you don't waste the money spent on the plan. The "free food" mentality is definitely the downfall of many college students during their freshman year.*

Competing Appetites

Even if your guy is evolved enough not to so much as flip through the *Sports Illustrated* swimsuit edition or glance at the Victoria's Secret window display in the mall, he can sabotage you in other ways. The danger with this kind of guy is that he likes to eat (and drink) and he wants you to join him at every bite.

No matter how many hours you spend at the gym and how few your boyfriend does, you cannot eat from the same plate, mouthful for mouthful. Sharing food is fine, as long as he eats two-thirds and you eat one-third. It's the gender differences that regulate height, lean body mass, and hormones that have given men a decided advantage at the table. Simply because they are male, they can stay in pretty good shape while eating like a locomotive and exerting very minimal amounts of energy. Women, on the other hand, must constantly tame their appetites and tone their muscles just to be entitled to a measly 1,600 calories a day.

If he wants your company at mealtime, and you enjoy his, be sure you have an equal voice in where you dine and how you split the bill. His goal will undoubtedly be to find large quantities of food at low prices. This often means buffets and all-you-can-eat restaurants. Not an easy place for you to figure out calories or portions. Your goal, on the other hand, should be to find good-quality food and an ample variety at reasonable prices. This may mean a diner or chain restaurant that has some calorie-conscious choices on its menu for you, right alongside all those belly-buster options for him.

The cardinal rule here is to hold your ground and not let him dictate all of the eating decisions. In fact, you can decline some of his invitations if it's just too much of a hassle to negotiate another limited-choice menu. Look at it this way: If he doesn't respect your preference for a portabello-topped veggie burger over his double-beef, cheese, and bacon burger, or your pasta primavera over his sausage-and-cheese lasagna, he may not be the guy for you anyway.

Feeding Your Emotions

If you are in the habit of reaching for something to eat every time you *feel* anything—happy, sad, excited, angry, lonely—it's time to change your mental health plan. You can't afford to spend the rest of the semester or the rest of your life medicating your feelings with food. There are way too many things over which you have no control and far too many feelings that can sneak up on you when you least expect them, to let this problem go untreated.

The treatment is to block your taste buds while you expand your mind. Refuse to eat for at least an hour after the emotional urge to eat hits you, and instead explore and unleash all those feelings. You can satisfy your emotional appetite by meditating or writing in a journal or talking to a friend or screaming in the shower. The goal here is to deal with the feelings and get comfortable with the way they come into and go out of your life. Eating to heighten or numb them can only lead to added pounds. Then you have to deal with that pain, too, which will be by the only way you know how namely, eating even more food. Get the picture?

Or if your emotions are starving for attention and the only remedy you can come up with is a pound of chocolate-covered pretzels, you need to institute the buddy system. Just as you were taught to never swim alone, you should also never ride an emotional roller coaster alone. Find a buddy whom you can trust, then empower her to accompany you on the rough rides and hold on tight. Tell her what you are feeling and what you are thinking of eating to deal with those feelings. Then let her help steer you back to safety.

Another convenient way to vent your emotions if your buddy isn't around is in a dieters' chat room. Keep the E-mail addresses in your Favorites file and go to it whenever grades, guys, or girlfriends screw up your day. The anonymous support and sisterhood in these on-line chats may be all that you need to curb your emotional eating and thwart the next mouthful leading to the freshman fifteen.

ENLARGE AND POST THIS!

QUICK-FIX FEEL-GOOD STRATEGIES TO COMBAT SABOTAGE

Rather than eat or drink to improve your spirits, spend a few bucks to pamper yourself. Whether flush with funds or down to your last few Abe Lincolns, there is something below to help make your day without overextending your caloric account.

BIG BUCKS	**BABY BUCKS**
Manicure	Nail polish
Facial	Lipstick
Pedicure	Socks
Haircut	Hair clip
Exfoliation	Eyebrow waxing
Massage	Yoga class
Spa treatment	Bubble bath
Concert ticket	Movie ticket
Cashmere sweater	Gap T-shirt
Leather boots	Funky sandals
Good jewelry	Faux jewelry
Bed comforter	Pillowcase

Metabolism Is Destiny

Cohabitation, as in dorm life, is a great place to learn about sharing and camaraderie. You may realize you like Mississippi blues after hearing it drift out of the room down the hall every night during your first six weeks on campus. You could become a regular at the foreign-film festival with the girls in your quad from Quebec. Your menstrual cycle may synchronize with that of your suitemates after living together for just two months. But you will also discover that no matter how much time you spend with another person, you cannot adopt her metabolism.

Sabotage can strike in the most unlikely places, and one of the deadliest is in the form of a friend who can eat whatever she wants and not gain weight. At least not now, anyway. You know who these people are and you must envy them, not emulate them. Whatever you do, do not try to convince yourself that because you are the same age and height as some people, wear the same size, and have the same tastes as they do, that you can eat the same amount of food they eat. There is no correlation here *at all*.

Keep one eye on the scale and the other on the mirror at all times if you spend any significant amount of time with someone who has one of these racehorse metabolisms. What she eats is abnormal and unfair. There is nothing you can do about it, so don't even bother trying to figure it out. Just be grateful you get to learn all about sensible eating and regular exercise while you're in college learning everything else that might be useful to you later in life.

✺ *MARISA:*
I knew it was better to either eat small portions throughout the day or just three balanced meals—my problem was, I did both. Whenever anyone else was eating, I joined in.

✺ *MARCHELLE:*
When I was out with my friends I would overindulge and wake up feeling disgusted. I finally realized that most of my friends were athletes and could get away with it because they burned more calories exercising.

Your poor friend is going to have to tackle all of these weight-control issues once she is older, say, in her late twenties, when her metabolism slows down. By that time, her voracious appetite will be so unregulated, she's going to have a much tougher time learning to count calories and measure portions, if she can deal with it at all. Your revenge will come at your ten-year college reunion. She'll be the one who looks least like her college picture.

Other People's Problems

Friends, family, and acquaintances with sluggish metabolisms can also sabotage you. They just go about it in more underhanded ways than their eat-everything-in-sight counterparts. Here's a vocabulary list of the ways their problems can ruin your self-control.

Jealousy = to resent, covet, envy

Someone who has not figured out how to measure out a cup of rigatoni from the pasta bar or stay on the elliptical machine in the fitness center for 30 minutes so she can burn off the 300 calories in that pasta is certainly not going to be thrilled to see you succeed. This is someone who will take as many hostages as she can when headed for the 24-hour mini-mart on the first night of finals week. And though she may sound like a friend when she says, *"I'll treat at the House of Pancakes for the Tuesday morning all-you-can-eat $2.99 special,"* she's not. Anyone who even mentions the words *pancakes* and *all-you-can-eat* in the same sentence should be looked at as suspect. This is sabotage with maple syrup dripping all over it.

Trifling = petty, paltry, irrelevant

Watch out for people who are constantly griping about the small, meaningless, insignificant stuff. These whiners and complainers can build up enough self-pity to feel entitled to a big payoff, and you never know when they're going to collect. Then, all of a sudden, someone's bad hair day becomes your diet disaster as she bursts into your dorm room to announce, *"I couldn't go to class because my hair was frizzy, so I baked some brownies."* This is the kind of sabotage you never see coming, so keep your door locked if it's humid outside.

Impetuous = rash, hasty, reckless

Even if you carefully make a shopping list and avoid the temptation aisles in the supermarket, there's always a chance someone else on the floor couldn't suppress her high-caloric cravings. And when others yield to their weaknesses, they do not go down alone. Their form of sabotage may sound like this: *"I just went downtown to get my nails done and when I passed the Italian bakery I saw a sign that said cannoli were on sale two for one, so I got us a dozen to share."* Immediately look for eleven other people to help her out of her dilemma and get the heck out of the building as fast as you can.

Rapacious = greedy, gluttonous, insatiable

Some people are very enthusiastic no matter what they are doing. They make the most mundane events seem exciting and can draw you into their hyperstimulated state just by saying "Let's go!" But if the invitation is to join such a friend for something to eat, decline the offer. If you don't, you will be caught up in a feeding frenzy with someone who doesn't know when to quit. She makes eating a sporting event and you can't afford to play at her game, let alone be a spectator. So when you hear, *"Let's rent a movie and get some marshmallows and stuff so we can make S'mores and Rice Krispies treats and hot chocolate,"* break out the books and head for the library.

Self-Inflicted Sabotage

You could easily avoid all this interference with your eating and exercise objectives for the next four years if you live alone and take correspondence courses so other people's problems can't entrap you. Yet even if you could do that, you would still have to face your own saboteurs—your personal explosives with your finger on the detonator. There is no hiding from them. So recognize your vulnerabilities and learn to defeat them. You may find that your GPA goes up while your weight goes down, because the same traits control success in both!

Laziness = idleness, apathy, slothfulness

If you have ever been accused of being lazy or are willing to admit that it is difficult to motivate yourself to do anything you know you should do, you're facing some big challenges as you fight the freshman fifteen. Counting calories and controlling portion sizes while getting regular exercise and passing your first-semester courses is a lot of hard work. Laziness just won't cut it and must be overcome—soon. So get organized, set priorities, focus on completing what you set out to do each day, and end the lame excuses.

Procrastination = to postpone, delay, or suspend

This is right up there with laziness and cannot be tolerated if you care at all about what size suit you'll be wearing when you go on your first job interview. Certain things must get done each and every day in order to keep those first 5 pounds from finding your particular seat in the Intro to Psych lecture hall and taking up space in your jeans. In fact, if you're paying attention to those lectures, you will soon realize you can't get what you want in life simply by wishing for it. You have been blessed with free will; now use it.

Trepidation = fear, misgivings, apprehension

Even the most ambitious and motivated person can be frozen in her tracks by fear of failure and fear of the unknown. The thought process goes something like this: "What if I follow all the rules and keep my weight under control and get good grades. Will I then know what I want to do with the rest of my life?" And the answer is "Who knows?" But it makes little sense to put your present dreams on hold due to uncertainty about whether or not they will make your future dreams come true. Get over it and get on with it because those extra pounds can sneak up on you quicker than you think.

Insomnia = sleeplessness, restlessness, agitation

You will leave college with countless fond memories, but none will have to do with how great the sleeping conditions were. In fact, you may earn your degree and not be able to recall ever having slept at all in the four to five years you spent completing the task. Consider this a surefire way to put on a pound a week your first semester. Here's how.

✹ *MARISA:*
I would always feel bad after a small splurge, so I would keep on going and just make myself feel worse. That's the story of my life with chocolate and ice cream.

✹ *MARCHELLE:*
After eating and drinking too much, I'd wake up feeling like a truck ran over my head. Then if I tried to go without eating for a day, I would splurge again later on. I finally realized that that wasn't working.

In your effort to stay awake around the clock due to demands of endless partying and studying, you will need more and more food to keep you going. Caffeine alone won't sustain you through the wee hours, night after night. You'll need sugars and simple carbohydrates to periodically jolt you into wakefulness, then high-protein, high-fat foods like cheeseburgers and fries to fuel you for the longer hauls. Feeding your body more and more calories when it is longing just for one good night's sleep is a way to wake up a whole lot fatter than you were before you finally nodded off.

Now you know all that you need to keep yourself emotionally on track. But you also need to run the track, or ride the stationary bicycle, or climb the step machine, or kick-box on the gym floor to keep yourself moving one step ahead of the freshman fifteen. Read on to find out how to win that race, too.

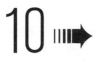

an extra-credit
course in exercise

U NLESS you are attending college on an athletic scholarship or you are majoring in dance with a minor in recreation, you're probably not getting enough physical activity (aka exercise). The only muscle you are likely to be using on a regular basis at all is your brain, and it burns very few calories per hour no matter how difficult the course load.

> ✺ *MARISA:*
> *I was so active in sports and dance lessons while in high school, I never went to a gym to work out. Once I hit college, it was hard to get motivated to go. When I did, it was more of a social thing—I don't think I broke a sweat.*
>
> ✺ *MARCHELLE:*
> *My school's gym facilities were surprisingly nice. I found it was a bit of a social hangout, so I actually went more often once I found I had all this free time in the afternoon. It was also a great way to meet guys.*

Fortunately, your campus is an oasis for physical activity and fitness opportunities. The goal of this chapter is to be sure you discover them all and learn to take secret delight in the fact that you have to walk a mile and a half uphill to your chemistry lab. And with that in mind the new dress code when leaving for class should be: sneakers.

Body Composition, or "You Are What You Eat"

The nutrients found in foods that are vital to our survival fall into six classes. The first is water, the most abundant nutrient found in foods and the one most essential to human life. Next in predominance are the energy- (or calorie-) yielding nutrients in foods: the carbohydrates, proteins, and fats. They also have important roles in building and maintaining body parts over a lifetime. Then in smaller but equally significant amounts are the nutrients classified as vitamins and minerals.

6 Major Nutrients Found in Food
1. Water
2. Protein
3. Fat
4. Carbohydrates
5. Vitamins
6. Minerals

It should come as no surprise that the very same nutrients we consume from the plants and animals we eat also make up the human body. Just like our food, human beings are composed primarily of water. The weight of the body is 55 to 60 percent water. The next major chunk of your weight is made up of fat. A healthy percentage of body fat is between 20 and 24 percent for women and 16 and 20 percent for men. Don't bother trying to fight this difference, girls; the higher fat content in a woman's body is due to the padding needed to protect the reproductive organs. When that percentage gets too low, as in the low teens for women, you stop menstruating and have a whole host of other problems as a result.

A more important place to make up the difference is in muscle mass. The muscles, which include all major organs and other lean tissue, such as red blood cells, contribute from 10 to 20 percent of a woman's weight. This is typically a higher percentage in males, even if they don't work out, because testosterone makes muscles and males have more of it. But physically active women *can* get their percentage of lean muscle mass into the high teens if they regularly find their way to the gym and move some metal.

Minerals found in the skeleton, like calcium and phosphorus, account for the next portion of body weight, with smaller amounts of minerals also located in teeth (fluoride), red blood cells (iron), muscles (magnesium), and cellular fluids (sodium, potassium). The total mineral weight of the body is about 6 to 8 percent.

This number varies depending on how dense the bones become as a result of the constant stress on the skeleton from heavy work or exercise. Genetic makeup also determines the degree of bone density, which is why some women are more prone to diseases like osteoporosis; their bones are simply smaller and more easily fractured.

The remaining 1 to 3 percent of body weight is made up of stored and circulating carbohydrates (muscle glycogen and blood glucose) and stored or circulating vitamins (vitamins A and D in the liver, vitamins B_1 and B_2 in enzymes).

To put all this in perspective, here is what the body of a 125-pound woman is made of:

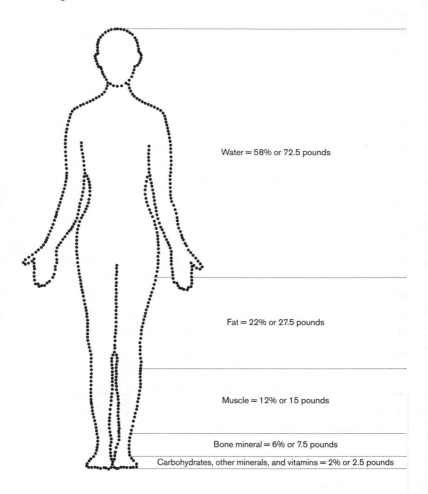

Water = 58% or 72.5 pounds

Fat = 22% or 27.5 pounds

Muscle = 12% or 15 pounds

Bone mineral = 6% or 7.5 pounds

Carbohydrates, other minerals, and vitamins = 2% or 2.5 pounds

The relevance of all this is that no matter how far you ran on the cross-country team in high school, or how many laps you swam in your summer job as a lifeguard, or how high the number of ab crunches you did every night on your bedroom floor last year, you do not get to keep the fat-to-muscle ratio you once had if you don't keep up the fat-burning, muscle-building workouts.

Your body composition will continually shift as a result of changes in the type and amount of physical activity you get. That means the more you sit and the less you move, the more your flesh is going to jiggle around when you do move. Body composition also changes with age so that no matter how vigilant you are about keeping that flesh firm, you've got to ratchet it up a notch every year just to stay ahead of the decline in metabolism that accompanies each birthday and can increase the jiggle factor.

Your time in college should serve as a training period for your lifelong commitment to regular fitness for the simple reason that if you can get it done there, you can get it done anywhere. Your erratic schedule, overwhelming course work, distracting extracurricular activities, and exhausted body need to learn to toe the line *now*, before real life sets in. Because then you will have to deal with a demanding job, a daily commute, monthly bills, complicated relationships, and an older body.

✳ *MARISA:*
My school provided tons of recreational classes, everything from yoga to martial arts. I found it boring to run on a treadmill, so I took advantage of these more creative workouts.

✳ *MARCHELLE:*
The classes offered at my school's gym were taught by other students and were free. I was surprised at what a great workout they were.

Forget willpower, girls, you'll need discipline to get this job done. It's not called "working" out for nothing. If you can think of it as a job and do it because you're being paid to do it, you might find the reserves you need to get it done. And the payoff is a stable weight through college and beyond, with a bonus package of toned muscles.

Your Exercise Objectives

The biggest misconception people have about their workouts is the notion that as long as they are doing something on a regular basis, that's good enough. Please pay attention here, girls, because a "good enough" attitude about exercise is not necessarily good or enough.

When it comes to really getting results from your workouts, it helps to think of your body as a farm. A farmer has to rotate what crops are planted in each patch of land and allow it to go fallow, or unplanted, some seasons in order to be rewarded with abundant harvests year after year. If she doesn't, she will have to do much more work tilling the soil and fighting the weeds for a less than lush crop yield.

Your muscles also need different toning and strength-building exercises to produce the best results from swimsuit season to downhill-skiing season. Doing the same workout week after week, month after month, will not keep all six hundred muscles in your body in shape and will actually yield fewer and fewer results the more you continue doing the same old thing.

On a farm there are also many chores that have to be done every day regardless of the weather or where you spent the previous night. Chickens certainly can't open the feedbag with their tiny beaks and cows won't start milking themselves, either, just because you'd rather sleep in.

If you think of your requirement for some type of daily exercise as a chore you really cannot neglect or the whole farm will fall apart, you may realize you do have the time and the means to do something every day to help keep yourself in shape. This is the one job in life you can't delegate to someone else or pay another person to do for you, no matter how much money you have. There are simply no acceptable excuses, so get up and start moving!

The goals for a well-tended body are to incorporate activities into your daily routines that develop these three areas of your fitness profile:

◆ Flexibility
◆ Stamina
◆ Strength

There are many options within each area, and the more you vary what you do, the better you'll look and feel.

Flexibility

The benefits of having flexible joints and muscles are that you can:

◆ Move more gracefully in your own body
◆ Maintain balance and posture more naturally
◆ Reduce the chances of suffering injuries from accidents and falls
◆ Prevent the pain and disability of arthritis

Stretching exercises and movements are the best way to remain flexible. Stretching puts the main joints of your body through their full range of motion while lengthening and loosening the muscles attached to those joints. Stretching should make you feel relaxed because it is done slowly, at your own pace, and is a completely noncompetitive activity.

Each stretching position should be held for 10 to 20 seconds, while taking full, even breaths throughout. Bouncing and jerky movements are not recommended, nor is any movement that causes pain and cannot be comfortably maintained for the 10-to-20-second count. It helps to try to visualize the muscle you are stretching while performing flexibility exercises and gently increase the contraction or extension to the point of mild tension—but never to the point where it causes pain.

Before a workout, it is always desirable to stretch the particular muscle group or part of your body that will be engaged in the physical activity you are about to perform. This targeted stretching helps to make the muscle more limber and directs blood flow to it, thus delivering needed oxygen.

Many forms of yoga provide a perfect way to gain the benefits of stretching and flexibility. Check out the classes available on campus to find one that fits into your schedule, and sign up immediately. The meditation portion will also help with stress management and craving control.

There are also many basic stretch routines you can learn from manuals and videos. No matter how limited the space you are confined to or how short the time you have, there are stretches you can do there and then. For example, stretches can be done while seated in a chair. Try them when studying or listening to long lectures or riding in a car. There are stretches that can be done using readily available props like towels and walls, ideally suited when drying off after a shower. Other stretches require nothing more than the area you take up when lying on the floor, best attempted after vacuuming.

✷ *MARCHELLE:*

I would arrange my schedule so all my classes were on Tuesdays and Thursdays, then I had plenty of time the other three days for some physical activity. My best friend and I would meet one day a week to play racquetball. Since neither of us knew how to play, it was a very demanding workout!

✷ *MARISA:*

I taped yoga, kick-boxing, and tai chi classes from television and would do them while doing my laundry. Once a week my friends and I would get together for a video workout, which was a lot of fun and much more motivational.

Stamina

The benefits of endurance training are:

- Muscles produce energy more efficiently so that you can do more with less effort
- You burn more calories when you can exercise for extended periods of time
- You can eat more without gaining weight
- The heart and lungs become stronger and life expectancy is extended

The heart is a muscle like any other in your body and can be conditioned to grow bigger and stronger through regular exercise. But to increase endurance, or the ability to do more work over longer periods of time with less effort, the circulatory system must also be conditioned so that it can carry all the blood and fresh oxygen to the cells as efficiently as possible.

Aerobic exercise is the best way to develop both the heart and the circulation—or cardiovascular system—to increase your endurance and help you feel more energetic. You should be able to get through each day feeling strong and vigorous so that you can do whatever you want to without copping out because you're too tired, too lazy, or too weak. Sound familiar?

That can happen even when you aren't overweight and don't appear to have excess flab on your body, but you are out of shape when it comes to cardiovascular conditioning. Then every little thing you do makes you feel more exhausted. Just to get out of bed, pull some clothes on, and walk across campus to your first class takes effort, and the harder your heart has to work, the sooner you will begin to feel fatigued. Then as the day wears on you will become more sluggish and look for any chance to sit instead of stand, stop instead of go, or sleep instead of do.

If you increase your aerobic activity, you will gain the stamina to do all of the things you need and want to get done each day, which can go a long way toward improving your mental outlook and reducing the stress of always falling behind in your deadlines.

Fitting in Fitness for Free

- ✦ Join an intramural team
- ✦ Take the stairs *every time*
- ✦ Walk the campus between classes
- ✦ Take a sports or fitness class
- ✦ Use a bike to do errands
- ✦ Get a job delivering newspapers on campus
- ✦ Sign up for fund-raising Walk-a-Thons
- ✦ Jog the track around the athletic fields

◆ Enter "field day" competitions between dorms
◆ Go to nightclubs to dance, not drink
◆ Sign up for any type of fun physical "marathon"—
  in-line skating, free-throw foul shooting, Hula-Hoops, tap
  dancing

Strength

Some of the key advantages to strength training are:

◆ Strong muscles have better shape, as in cut, definition,
  sculpting
◆ Posture is better when muscles are strong, giving a
  taller, more proportioned appearance
◆ Endurance, or aerobic capacity, is improved with strong
  muscles
◆ Muscles burn more calories than fat even when not
  in use
◆ Strong muscles protect bone density

Strength training is also called weight lifting, pumping
iron, and resistance exercise. It involves isolating and moving a
muscle against a weight or resistance that can be made heavier
and heavier. The weight of the resistance can vary using bar-
bells, dumbbells, and other exercise equipment and machines.
By varying the resistance, number of repetitions performed,
and frequency of training, you can get bigger, bulkier muscles
or longer and more shapely muscles.

Strength is not determined by size alone. Dancers and gym-
nasts are every bit as strong as football and hockey players.
They have different performance goals that determine how big
to build their muscles and how fast and flexible they have to be
as well. It is virtually impossible for a woman to build huge

muscles unless she really, really works at it. Of greater concern is creating a disproportioned figure due to overwork of some areas of the body and underdevelopment of others.

Another big advantage of continually building and maintaining your muscle mass is in the way it speeds up your metabolism. If you think of your muscles like the engine of a car, then you can imagine that your muscles are going to burn calories, or fuel, every time you start up the engine to go somewhere. The more muscles you have, or the bigger the engine in a car, the more fuel you're going to burn whether in motion or idle. It is estimated that every pound of lean muscle burns an additional 30 to 50 calories each day. That's a real bonus if you also happen to like to eat.

It also becomes more relevant when you realize that muscles naturally diminish with age. That means your metabolism is slowing down a little bit each year with each pound of muscle you lose. Then, even if you consume the same number of calories each day, you will gradually become fatter unless you work at replacing the lost muscle through a regular regimen of strength training. Here's how that looks, starting at age fourteen, when you are at your peak muscle mass.

⚹ MARISA:
I found I preferred activities that were fun and did not make me feel like I was working out. I took golf and tennis lessons and ballroom dancing, hip-hop, and salsa classes.

⚹ MARCHELLE:
I bought a little weight set that came in a briefcase so I could get in a quick workout anytime I wanted to. And if you have a VCR and a mat to throw on the floor, there are loads of videos you can do in a confined space.

Table 10.1

CHANGES IN MUSCLE-TO-FAT RATIO IN WOMEN WITH AGING

Without a deliberate increase in muscle-toning exercises throughout her life, a woman's body composition can change in the following ways even if she continues to consume the same number of calories from one decade to the next, due to the effects of a slower metabolism and a loss of lean muscle mass.

Age	14	20	30	40	50
Body Weight (lbs.)	120	126	136	146	156
Muscle (lbs.)	48	45	40	35	30
Percent Muscle	40%	36%	29%	24%	19%
Fat (lbs.)	20	29	44	59	74
Percent Fat	17%	23%	32%	40%	47%

WEIGHING THE OPTIONS

You are never far from a good resistance workout when you consider that moving your own body weight is a great way to do strength training. In the space of your dorm room you can any of the following:

BACK AND CHEST	LEGS AND BUTT	ABDOMINALS	ARMS AND SHOULDERS
Basic push-ups	Leg lifts	Basic crunches	Dips
Deltoid push-ups	Squats	Diagonal crunches	Curls*
Chin-ups	Lunges	Elevated crunches	Lateral raises*
Pull-ups	Leg extensions	Diamond crunches	Elbow presses*

For the price of your tuition, you are undoubtedly entitled to the use of the "fitness laboratory," or gym or weight room on campus. Find it and use it for a more versatile weight-training program.

* A one-pound can of vegetables can initially be used for light weights.

Physical Fitness Vocabulary List

Abdominals: Several specific muscles that form the front, sides, and back of the middle body giving shape to the torso and support to the spine. There is no one movement that can engage all of the muscles that define this area, and no amount of abdominal exercise that can reduce excessive fat storage in the belly.

Abductor: The *outer* thigh muscles, which run from the top of the hip down the side of the thigh.

Adductor: The *inner* thigh muscles, which run along the inside of the upper leg.

Aerobic exercise: Any activity during which the working muscles must be supplied with extra oxygen to meet the energy demands of the workload. These activities usually make you breathe harder and more deeply to deliver the additional oxygen to the muscles, but they should not leave you breathless. Aerobic activity should be done at a level you can sustain for longer periods of time with steady, even breathing. The more aerobic activity one does, the more efficient this oxygen delivery system becomes and the more capable the muscles are of producing the energy they need by drawing on stored fat as a fuel.

Anaerobic exercise: Exercise done at a high intensity, and usually for short periods, where the energy needs of the muscles cannot be met by the aerobic system. Instead, energy is produced without oxygen using the fuels found directly in the muscle (glycogen, lactic acids, protein). Anaerobic exercises can help increase muscle mass, but they are not as effective as aerobic exercise in depleting fat stores.

Basal metabolic rate (BMR): The minimum amount of energy required to sustain the vital functions of the body in a waking state. BMR declines as we age but can be raised by increasing the muscle mass of the body.

Biceps: A two-part muscle in the front of the upper arm.

Calisthenics: Any exercise that is done in rhythmic repetitions, usually in one place, like jumping jacks, but not for long enough periods of time to make it fully aerobic. While not as effective in burning fat reserves, calisthenics can be useful in building strength and endurance.

Cellulite: Most people recognize it when they see it, but from a scientific point of view cellulite doesn't exist. It is nothing more than fat cells that, on some people's bodies, form dimples. Think of them as "fat freckles."

Gluteus maximus: The muscle that lies beneath and gives shape to the buttocks.

Hamstring: A three-part muscle that forms the back of the thigh along with the gluteus maximus.

Heart rate: The waves of pressure, or pulse, that can be manually counted on the artery on the thumb side of the wrist, at the side of the temple, or along the side of the trachea (Adam's apple) in the neck. The heart rate or pulse rate are used to measure and monitor levels of exercise exertion.

Interval training: Short bursts of high-intensity activity, interspersed with periods of rest or lower-level activity, such as the intermittent fast and slow programs on treadmills. The longer the periods of intense activity, the greater the aerobic benefits.

Isometric exertion: An activity in which muscles push against a fixed resistance, such as pressing the palms of the hands together as hard and long as possible. During these exercises the muscles expend energy and build in strength and size, but they do not produce movement and have no aerobic effect.

Isotonic exertion: Any exercise in which a particular muscle group contracts repeatedly at controlled or variable speeds against a constant resistance, such as in lifting weights or doing sit-ups. These exercises can build muscle strength and size, but have little aerobic effect unless several sets of the exercises are done at a fast pace without resting in between.

Quadriceps: A four-part muscle that shapes the front of the thigh and supplies the power for any forward movement, like walking.

"Reps" or repetitions: The same exercise repeated a certain number of times, or "reps," before stopping to rest or do another exercise.

Sets: Performing a single exercise for a certain number of reps, then resting and doing it again for a second or third set of that same exercise.

Triceps: A three-part muscle making up most of the back of the upper arm.

Finding Time for Fitness

Now you know that in addition to the 15 credits you're carrying and the 1,500 calories a day you're trying to keep track of, you've also got to do at least 15 minutes of daily stretching plus 15 minutes of strength training and another 30 minutes of aerobic activity to fight the freshman fifteen. "How's a girl supposed to get it all done and still have time for fun?" you ask. It's not easy, but it is doable.

The trick is in multitasking, or doing two or more things at once. You might want to start by wearing a pedometer, which can keep track of how many miles you walk in the course of your daily activities. For most people with an average stride length, you'll take 2,000 steps to walk 1 mile. Since that's probably not in one uninterrupted jaunt, it will not be as aerobic as a brisk 15-minute walk on a treadmill, and therefore will not have the same calorie-burning, endurance-building benefits. But if you walk enough, it does add up to those same benefits. You will have to log in about 10,000 steps a day, or 5 miles on the pedometer, to meet this fitness requirement.

You can also incorporate stretching moves into your sedentary time, while watching TV or whenever you are hanging around "waiting" for anybody. Do a series of muscle contractions and releases to make better use of your time in lines and on hold. In fact, if you make it a practice never to sit down while talking on the phone, you can have remarkably tighter abs and butt. Here's how:

Keeping the phone in one hand, suck in your stomach to contract the abdominals and hold for a count of 10. Then slowly release and repeat for a total of 8 reps. Now squeeze the butt together and hold for 10 seconds, then release and repeat for 8 reps. If you're still on the phone, do another set. After 3 sets, you can move on to work your calves.

Lean against a wall for balance and rise up on your toes. Hold the position for 10 seconds, then slowly lower yourself and repeat for 8 reps. Then rock back on your heels and stretch your toes upward for a count of 10. Lower and complete 8 reps each, for 1 set. Keep going for a total of 3 sets, time permitting.

Another way to double up your exercise time is by combining upper and lower body exercises in a weight-training session. For example, bicep curls can be done while lunging and front arm lifts while squatting. Check out the websites below for more quickie exercise combos.

On-Line Resources

www.digiwalker.com: site for the Yamax Digi-Walker pedometer.

www.nutristrategy.com: information about nutrition and exercise plus a free newsletter subscription.

11 ⅢⅢ➡

recipes for dorm-room dining

I F you've stocked your pantry with the provisions itemized in chapter 4, you should be able to whip up any of the recipes provided here and steer clear of all those unwanted calories tempting you all over campus. You can customize these recipes to suit your tastes and preferences by adding more or different vegetables and seasonings or by substituting some reduced-fat or fat-free products where low-fat ones are mentioned.

The nutritional information given for each recipe is based on the use of the ingredients described in them. Your actual nutrient content may vary if you make substitutions.

Out-the-Door Breakfasts

☼ TASTY TOAST

¹/₂ cup low-fat cottage cheese
2 tablespoons sugar-free jam
2 slices of light wheat bread, toasted
¹/₂ cup sliced fresh fruit of your choice

Mix together the cottage cheese and the jam, then spread it on the toast and top with the sliced fruit.

Calories: 260 / Food groups: 1 grain, 1 dairy, ½ fruit + 50 extra calories

❄ CREAMY MELON BOWL

1 cup chopped melon of your choice
½ cup fat-free vanilla yogurt
2 tablespoons raisins
3 tablespoons low-fat high-fiber cereal or granola

Place the melon in the bottom of a bowl, then layer with the yogurt, raisins, and cereal or granola.

Calories: 200 / Food groups: ½ grain, ½ dairy, 2 fruit

❄ BURRITO TO GO

2 egg whites or ¼ cup Egg Beaters
1 6" low-fat wheat tortilla
1 low-fat cheese single
2 tablespoons salsa

Spray a frying pan with nonstick cooking spray, place it over medium heat, and scramble the egg whites or Egg Beaters. Microwave the tortilla with the cheese for 1 minute, then roll up with the salsa and eggs inside.

Calories: 200 / Food groups: 1 grain, ½ dairy, 1 meat

❄ CRAN-BANANA BLENDER

½ cup chopped banana
½ cup ice
½ cup orange juice
⅓ cup cranberry juice

Blend all of the ingredients in a blender and enjoy. You can add some fresh or frozen berries if you have them on hand.

Calories: 150 / Food groups: 2½ fruit

POWER TOAST

2 slices light wheat bread, toasted

2 tablespoons peanut butter

1 low-fat cheese single

Spread 1 slice of warm toast with peanut butter, then add the cheese and top with the other slice of toast, then melt.

Calories: 320 / Food groups: 1 grain, ½ dairy, 2 meat

NUTTY MORNING SALAD

1 tablespoon honey

2 tablespoons walnuts (or whatever nuts you have on hand)

½ cup chopped apple

¼ cup low-fat cottage cheese

2 tablespoons raisins

1 cup mixed greens or any kind of lettuce

Drizzle the honey over the walnuts and stir to combine. Mix the apple, cottage cheese, and raisins together. Spoon over lettuce and top with wet walnuts.

Calories: 260 / Food groups: ½ dairy, 1 meat, 1½ fruit, ½ veg + 60 extra calories

EARLY EGG SCRAMBLE

¼ cup diced tomato or salsa

2 slices of your favorite low-fat lunch meat cut into pieces

2 egg whites or ½ cup Egg Beaters

2 tablespoons fat-free milk

1 low-fat cheese single
Tabasco or other hot sauce to taste

Spray a frying pan with nonstick cooking spray and put over medium heat. Add the tomatoes or salsa and meat and cook for five minutes. Mix egg whites or Egg Beaters with the milk and pour into the pan over the tomato and meat. Stir and cook until almost firm, then add the cheese and Tabasco.

Calories: 125 / Food groups: ½ dairy, ½ meat, ½ veg

✸ BREAKFAST SAMMIE

1 egg or ½ cup Egg Beaters
2 slices light wheat bread, toasted
1 low-fat cheese single

Spray a frying pan with nonstick cooking spray and put over medium-high heat. Fry the eggs or Egg Beaters while the bread is toasting. Place the eggs and cheese on 1 piece of toast, then top with the other piece of toast for a sammie.

Calories: 225 / Food groups: 2 grain, ½ dairy, 1 meat

✸ FRUIT SALAD COMBO

½ cup chopped apple
½ cup chopped banana
½ cup chopped orange
1 tablespoon lemon juice
½ cup of fat-free vanilla yogurt
½ cup low-fat cottage cheese

Mix the fruits together. Then alternate layers of yogurt, fruit, and cottage cheese and repeat until all ingredients are used; or just mush everything together and eat.

Calories: 200 / Food groups: 1 dairy, 1½ fruit

One-Handed Sammies

A sammie is a sandwich, a meal you can eat with one hand!

✳ TOASTED CHEESE SAMMIE
1 tablespoon low-fat mayonnaise
2 slices light wheat bread, toasted
2 slices low-fat cheese singles
4 thin slices tomato

Spread mayonnaise on each piece of toast, then top each with a slice of cheese and 2 slices tomato. Place in a toaster oven for 1 minute, until the cheese melts. Put the 2 halves together for a sammie.

Calories: 235 / Food groups: 1 grain, 1 dairy, ½ veg, 1 fat

✳ EVERYTHING SAMMIE
2 thin slices of onion
2 thin slices of tomato
¼ cup black beans, drained
1 low-fat cheese single
2 slices low-fat ham
2 slices light wheat bread, toasted
¼ cup shredded lettuce
2 tablespoons vinegar

Layer onion, tomato, beans, cheese, and ham on one slice of toast. Top with lettuce and vinegar, then press other piece of toast on top for a sammie.

Calories: 200 / Food groups: 1 grain, ½ dairy, 1 meat, ½ veg

✳ CHICKEN TERIYAKI SAMMIE

$^1/_4$ cup chopped onion
2 teaspoons teriyaki sauce
$^3/_4$ cup canned chunk white chicken
1 slice light wheat bread, toasted

Spray a frying pan with nonstick cooking spray and place over medium heat. Cook the onion with the teriyaki sauce until the onion is soft. Add the chicken and cook for 2 more minutes. Spoon over the toast.

Calories: 150 / Food groups: ¹⁄₂ grain, 2 meat, ¹⁄₄ veg

✳ TUNA-WITH-THE-WORKS SAMMIE

$^1/_2$ cup canned water-packed tuna, drained
$^1/_2$ cup fresh or canned sliced mushrooms, drained
$^1/_4$ cup quartered canned artichoke hearts, drained
$^1/_4$ cup chopped celery
1 tablespoon low-fat mayonnaise
1 teaspoon mustard
1 tablespoons relish
2 slices light wheat bread, toasted

Mix all of the ingredients together and spread on the 2 pieces of toast for a sammie.

Calories: 275 / Food groups: 1 grain, 1 meat, 1 veg, 1 fat

✳ TURKEY-CRAN SAMMIE

1 thin slice jellied cranberry sauce
2 slices light wheat bread, toasted
2 teaspoons mustard
4 slices low-fat turkey breast
2 lettuce leaves
2 tomato slices

Spread the cranberry sauce on one piece of toast and the mustard on the other, then top 1 slice with the remaining ingredients. Put other slice on top for a sammie.

Calories: 200 / Food groups: 1 grain, ½ meat, ½ veg + 50 extra calories

✵ TASTY CHICKEN MELT SAMMIE

½ cup canned chunk white chicken
¼ cup chopped canned artichoke hearts, drained
2 tablespoons chopped onion
1 slice light wheat bread, toasted
1 low-fat cheese single

Combine chicken, artichoke hearts, and onion. Place the mixture on the toast, then top with cheese. Microwave for 1½ minutes for an open-faced sammie.

Calories: 200 / Food groups: ½ grain, ½ dairy, 1 meat, ½ veg

✵ MINI CHICKEN BURRITO

½ cup chunk white chicken
¼ cup salsa
¼ cup black beans, drained
1 6" low-fat wheat tortilla
1 low-fat cheese single

Combine the chicken, salsa, and black beans, then spread the mixture on the tortilla. Tear up the cheese and scatter over it. Microwave for 1½ minutes. Roll up for a sammie.

Calories: 300 / Food groups: 1 grain, ½ dairy, 1½ meat, ½ veg

✵ ASIAN DE-LITE SAMMIE

½ cup light tofu, drained and cubed
1 teaspoon reduced-sodium soy sauce

1 teaspoon teriyaki sauce
2 slices of light wheat bread, toasted

Put tofu in a microwave-safe bowl and coat with the soy and teriyaki sauces. Microwave for two minutes, then spoon the mixture over 1 piece of toast and top with the other for a sammie.

Calories: 200 / Food groups: 1 grain, 1 meat

❂ TURKEY WRAP

1 tablespoon low-fat cream cheese
$1/4$ cup salsa
1 6" low-fat wheat tortilla
2 slices low-fat turkey breast
$1/2$ cup fresh or canned spinach leaves
1 low-fat cheese single

Mix together the cream cheese and salsa, then spread the mixture over the softened tortilla. Top with the turkey, spinach, and cheese single. Roll up the tortilla for a sammie.

Calories: 225 / Food groups: 1 grain, $1/2$ dairy, $1/4$ meat, 1 veg, 1 fat

❂ BARBECUE CHICKEN SAMMIE

$1/2$ cup canned chunk white chicken
$1/4$ cup chopped tomato
1 tablespoon barbecue sauce
1 tablespoon low-fat mayonnaise
2 slices light wheat bread, toasted

Mix together everything but the bread, then spread the mixture on 1 piece of toast and top with the other for a sammie.

Calories: 250 / Food groups: 1 grain, 1 meat, $1/4$ veg, 1 fat

No Cook, No-Mess Meals

✸ HUMMUS TOPPED BREAD

2 tablespoons hummus
1 slice light wheat bread, toasted
4 slices of your favorite fat-free lunch meat
$1/4$ cup diced tomato

Spread the hummus on the toast, top with the lunch meat, then add the tomato.

Calories: 150 / Food groups: $1/2$ grain, 1 meat, $1/4$ veg

✸ MINI PIZZA

$1/4$ cup pasta sauce
2 slices light white bread
4 low-fat white cheese singles
$1/4$ cup diced tomato

Spread the pasta sauce on the bread, then cover with the cheese and tomato slices. Microwave for 1 to 2 minutes to melt the cheese.

Calories: 275 / Food groups: 1 grain, 2 dairy, 1 veg

✸ SPRINGTIME SALAD

2 tablespoons vinegar
1 teaspoon honey
2 teaspoons lemon juice
2 cups fresh spinach or lettuce leaves
$1/2$ cup chopped oranges or mandarin oranges
in light syrup, drained
2 tablespoons sliced almonds

Mix the vinegar, honey, and lemon juice together to make the salad dressing. Combine the remaining ingredients and drizzle the dressing on top.

Calories: 230 / Food groups: 1 meat, 1 fruit, 2 veg + 20 extra calories

✵ SPICY CHICKEN SALAD

$1/2$ cup canned chunk white chicken
2 fat-free cheese singles, cut into small pieces
$1/4$ cup salsa
$1/4$ cup low-fat cottage cheese
2 cups shredded lettuce

Combine the chicken with the cheese pieces and the salsa. Microwave for 1 to 2 minutes, then add the cottage cheese. Spoon over the lettuce.

Calories: 275 / Food groups: $1^1/2$ dairy, 1 meat, 1 veg

✵ RANCH VEGGIE MIXER

1 cup cottage cheese
2 tablespoons low-fat ranch dressing
$1/4$ cup chopped celery
$1/4$ cup chopped carrots
$1/4$ cup chopped broccoli

Mix all of the ingredients together and eat up.

Calories: 275 / Food groups: 2 dairy, 1 veg, 1 fat

❊ CHINESE CHICKEN SALAD

¹/₂ cup canned chunk white chicken

¹/₄ cup chopped celery

2 tablespoons low-fat mayonnaise

1 teaspoon duck sauce

1 teaspoon mustard

2 cups lettuce, torn into small pieces

Mix all of the ingredients together and spoon over the lettuce.

Calories: 250 / Food groups: 2 meat, 1 veg, 2 fat

❊ SPICY MACHO NACHOS

18 to 20 low-fat baked tortilla chips

¹/₄ cup black beans, drained

2 low-fat cheese singles, cut into strips

3 tablespoons low-fat sour cream

¹/₄ cup salsa

Place the chips on a plate, then scatter the beans over them and top with the cheese strips. Microwave for 1¹/₂ minutes or until the cheese has melted. Top with the sour cream and salsa.

Calories: 325 / Food groups: 2 grain, 1 dairy, ¹/₂ meat, ¹/₂ veg, 1 fat

❊ COBB COMBO CHOPPED SALAD

2 hardboiled egg whites, chopped

2 cups chopped lettuce

2 slices of low-fat lunch meat, diced

2 low-fat cheese singles, sliced

¹/₄ cup chopped tomatoes

¹/₄ cup sliced fresh or canned mushrooms

2 tablespoons low-fat salad dressing of your choice

Mix all of the ingredients in a bowl and drizzle on your favorite salad dressing.

Calories: 275 / Food groups: 1 dairy, 1 meat, 2 veg, 1 fat

�֎ SOUTH-OF-THE-BORDER CHICKEN

$1/2$ cup canned chunk white chicken
$1/4$ cup black beans, drained
$1/4$ cup salsa
2 low-fat cheese singles
2 tablespoons low-fat sour cream

Mix all of the ingredients together in a bowl except for the sour cream and microwave for $1^1/2$ minutes. Top with the sour cream and enjoy it while it's hot.

Calories: 275 / Food groups: 1 dairy, $1^1/2$ meat, $1/2$ veg, 1 fat

Satisfying Anytime Snacks

✷ FIBER 'N FRUIT

$1/2$ cup chopped apple
$1/2$ cup fat-free vanilla yogurt
$1/2$ cup low-fat high-fiber cereal or granola

Mix it all together and enjoy.

Calories: 175 / Food groups: 1 grain, $1/2$ dairy, $1/2$ fruit

✵ FRUIT-TOPPED COTTAGE CHEESE

1 cup low-fat cottage cheese
$\frac{1}{2}$ cup chopped banana
1 tablespoon honey

Mix the cottage cheese with the banana, then drizzle the honey on top.

Calories: 275 / Food groups: 2 dairy, $\frac{1}{2}$ fruit + 60 extra calories

✵ ORANGE-NANA DRINK

1 cup orange juice
$\frac{1}{2}$ cup chopped banana
$\frac{1}{2}$ cup crushed ice

Blend together until smooth.

Calories: 150 / Food groups: 2$\frac{1}{2}$ fruit

✵ PINK CELERY

2 tablespoons low-fat cream cheese
2 teaspoons strawberry jam or fruit spread
3 celery sticks

Combine cream cheese with jam. Then spread the cream cheese in the center of the celery, cut into 3" pieces, and eat.

Calories: 100 / Food groups: 1 veg, 1 fat + 35 extra calories

✵ TANGY TOMATO SALAD

1 cup chopped tomato
$\frac{1}{4}$ cup diced onion
2 tablespoons low-fat French dressing
1 low-fat cheese single, cut into strips

Combine the tomato and the onion, then drizzle with the dressing and top with the cheese.

Calories: 140 / Food groups: 2 veg, ½ dairy, 1 fat

❈ CREAMY FROZEN FRUIT

1 cup grapes, frozen
1 cup fat-free raspberry yogurt

Mix together in a bowl and enjoy a healthy frozen snack.

Calories: 225 / Food groups: 1 dairy, 2 fruit

❈ CRUNCHY YOGURT BLEND

1 cup fat-free coffee yogurt
½ cup chopped frozen banana
4 tablespoons low-fat granola

Blend the yogurt and the banana together, then top with the granola. Enjoy this delicious snack with a spoon.

Calories: 200 / Food groups: ½ grain, 1 dairy, ½ fruit

❈ CITRUS DRIZZLE

1 tablespoon lemon juice
1 tablespoon honey
1 teaspoon cinnamon
½ cup grapefruit sections
½ cup orange sections or ½ cup canned mandarin oranges, drained

Mix the lemon juice, honey, and cinnamon together and microwave for thirty seconds, then drizzle over the grapefruit and orange sections.

Calories: 175 / Food groups: 2 fruit + 60 extra calories

✺ LUNCH MEAT ROLL-UPS

2 tablespoons low-fat cream cheese

2 tablespoons chopped celery

1 teaspoon Italian seasoning blend

1 teaspoon mustard

4 slices low-fat lunch meat

Mix all of the ingredients together except for the lunch meat. Spread the mixture on the lunch meat, then roll up each slice and enjoy.

Calories: 100 / Food groups: ½ meat, 1 fat

✺ NUTTER BUTTER BLEND

1 cup fat-free milk

1 tablespoon peanut butter

1 tablespoon honey

Place everything in a blender and puree until frothy.

Calories: 250 / Food groups: 1 dairy, 1 meat + 60 extra calories

Must-Have Desserts

✺ CHOCOLATE STRAWBERRY SENSATION

½ cup fat-free vanilla ice cream or frozen yogurt

2 tablespoons fat-free chocolate syrup

½ cup sliced strawberries

2 tablespoons crushed fat-free graham crackers or granola

Scoop the ice cream into a bowl, then top with the syrup, strawberries, and graham cracker crumbs.

Calories: 200 / Food groups: ¼ grain, ½ fruit, +150 extra calories

MONKEY SHAKE

$^1/_2$ cup fat-free frozen yogurt
1 cup fat-free milk
$^1/_2$ cup chopped banana
$^1/_2$ cup ice

Blend all of the ingredients together and pour into a glass.

Calories: 250 / Food groups: 1 dairy, $^1/_2$ fruit + 100 extra calories

FROZEN FRUIT SURPRISE

1 cup fat-free vanilla yogurt
$^1/_2$ cup chopped and drained apricots, pears,
or other canned fruit
2 tablespoons low-fat granola or other crunchy cereal

Blend all of the ingredients together and pour into a plastic cup. Freeze for at least 4 hours before eating.

Calories: 175 / Food groups: $^1/_4$ grain, 1 dairy, 1 fruit

BLUE SHAKE

$^3/_4$ cup fat-free milk
$^3/_4$ cup fat-free blueberry yogurt
$^1/_2$ cup frozen blueberries

Blend it all together until smooth.

Calories: 200 / Food groups: 1$^1/_2$ dairy, $^1/_2$ fruit

✲ SOY FRUIT PUDDING

$^{1}/_{2}$ cup light tofu
$^{1}/_{2}$ cup chopped fresh or canned fruit, drained
3 tablespoons water
$^{1}/_{2}$ package sugar-free instant chocolate pudding mix

Place all of the ingredients in a blender container and blend until smooth.

Calories: 250 / Food groups: 1 meat, $^{1}/_{2}$ fruit + 100 extra calories

✲ TROPICAL SUNRISE SHAKE

$^{1}/_{4}$ cup canned pineapple, drained
$^{1}/_{4}$ cup canned peaches, drained
1 cup fat-free lemon yogurt
$^{1}/_{2}$ cup ice

Blend all of the ingredients together in a blender.

Calories: 175 / Food groups: 1 dairy, 1 fruit

✲ PUDDING SENSATION

$^{1}/_{2}$ cup ready-to-eat fat-free chocolate pudding
$^{1}/_{4}$ cup chopped banana
2 tablespoons chopped pecans or other nuts
2 tablespoons raisins

Mix it all and eat up.

Calories: 275 / Food groups: 1 meat, $1^{1}/_{4}$ fruit + 100 extra calories

✲ PINEAPPLE PARADISE

$^{1}/_{2}$ cup fat-free vanilla ice cream or frozen yogurt
$^{1}/_{2}$ cup fat-free milk
$^{1}/_{2}$ cup canned crushed pineapple, drained

Blend all of the ingredients together in a blender for the perfect tropical shake.

Calories: 200 / Food groups: ½ milk, ½ fruit + 100 extra calories

✶ ISLAND-STYLE YOGURT WITH A CRUNCH

1 cup fat-free strawberry yogurt
¼ cup crushed pineapple, drained
¼ cup mandarin oranges, drained
2 tablespoons almonds or other nuts
1 dollop fat-free Cool Whip

Mix all of the ingredients together and top with Cool Whip.

Calories: 275 / Food groups: 1 dairy, 1 fruit, 1 mcat + 20 extra calories

✶ BANANA BOAT

½ cup sliced banana
½-inch-thick piece angel food cake
4 tablespoons fat-free Cool Whip
1 tablespoon sliced almonds or other nuts

Place the banana on the cake, then top with the Cool Whip and sprinkle with the almonds.

Calories: 250 / Food groups: ½ meat, ½ fruit + 150 extra calories

❄ SWEET TOOTH TOAST

1 slice light white bread, toasted
1 tablespoon low-fat cream cheese
1 teaspoon brown sugar
1 teaspoon cinnamon
1 tablespoon raisins

While the bread is toasting, mix the cream cheese with the brown sugar and cinnamon, then spread it on the warm bread and top with the raisins.

Calories: 120 / Food groups: ½ grain, ½ fruit, ½ fat + 25 extra calories

❄ FRUIT DIP

½ cup low-fat cottage cheese
2 tablespoons sugar-free strawberry jam
1 apple, sliced

Mix the cottage cheese and the jam until they are creamy or use a blender to combine. Dip the apple slices into this delicious sauce.

Calories: 200 / Food groups: 1 dairy, 1 fruit + 50 extra calories

about the authors

ROBYN FLIPSE has been a registered dietitian providing individual and group counseling for nutrition and eating disorders for more than twenty-five years. In her vast experience with children, teens, and adults, she has learned all of the reasons *why* people gain weight at different stages of the life cycle and how to both prevent it and reverse the pattern if it has already begun.

Her insight into the most common times for gaining weight and not losing it led her to write her first book, ***The Wedding Dress Diet.*** Now she is reaching out to young women who want to avoid the inevitable weight gain that can accompany their freshman year.

Flipse's professional expertise is complemented by the anecdotes of two sisters, MARISA and MARCHELLE BRADANINI, who share their own experiences of gaining weight once in college. They also created the fifty recipes that appear in the book—ones they used to get back to their original weights and to maintain them until they graduated.